FROM SUICIDAL TO
Serene

This book is dedicated to individuals young and old in this country who are suffering from physical and mental disease as well as emotional traumas, and to all the individuals who are healing sick individuals in any way such as functional medical doctors, psychologists, hypnotherapists, and therapists, etc.

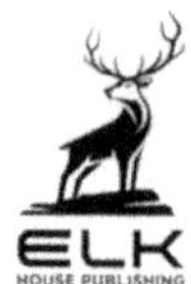

Contact information for Elk House Publishing: elkhousepublishing@gmail.com

ISBN: 979-8-9860045-0-1 (paperback)
ISBN: 979-8-9860045-1-8 (ebook)

Ordering Information:
Special discounts are available on quantity purchases by corporations, associations, and others. For details, contact elkhousepublishing@gmail.com

TABLE OF
Contents

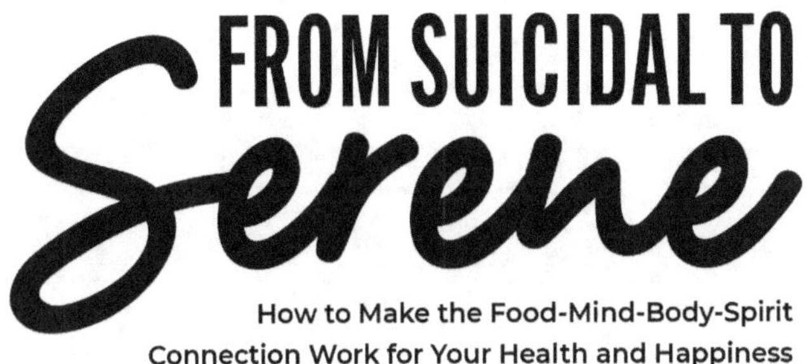

FROM SUICIDAL TO Serene

How to Make the Food-Mind-Body-Spirit
Connection Work for Your Health and Happiness

AMIR SIDDIQUI

Disclaimer

In sharing my experiences with you, my intimate personal experiences as well as experiences with the modalities and therapies I tried during my personal growth journey, my hope is to give you some kind of guidance to inspire you into your own personal growth journey. Although these are my individual experiences, I believe anyone can learn from them and improve their lives based on what I've been through. However, I have no relationship whatsoever with any brands or companies I mention in this book. Moreover, you should do your own research and use your own judgment prior to using any of these products or services. The information provided in this book is for information purposes only, and is for you to use at your own discretion.

INTRODUCTION

From Darkness to Light

From Darkness to Light

I used to suffer from frustration, jealousy, resentment, bitterness, hopelessness, anxiety, road rage, and anger. I expressed anger both passively and aggressively.

I also suffered from severe depression that eventually turned into suicidal tendencies for a year and a half. I had thoughts come and go so fast that my mind used to get tired. I couldn't focus on anything. I had been living life reacting to people, conditions, and circumstances.

It didn't take much to set me off. For instance, if another driver cut me off on the road, I would yell and honk at them. I would complain for 20 minutes about how mean people are to drive like that. I would ruin my own day over minor incidents, then do it all again the next day.

I lived life on autopilot for a long time. It felt like I had no control and that things were happening whether I wanted them to or not—but then everything changed.

The moment my life changed was shortly after I got married. I knew I would need to produce more income in order to support my wife and I. The income I was making at the time just wasn't enough. I didn't know it at the time, but as I began to pursue higher income options and avenues, this is also where I began my personal growth journey that eventually led me to discover a great, though invisible, power inside of myself.

Now I experience predominantly positive emotions of gratitude, joy, enthusiasm, serenity, pride, hope, faith, love, and peace. I move through my day with focus. My thoughts are under control. Has my life become perfect? Not at all. I still get annoyed if another driver cuts me off, but I usually get over it in a few minutes. It no longer ruins my whole day and I don't obsess over it.

I attract happier customers and people, but if and when I attract angry or negative customers and people, I deal with them assertively. I learned that I can't control anything outside of me and the only thing I have control over is how I respond to anything and everything.

Though I still have many challenges, I am now in control of my life, and I want to help you achieve what I have achieved.

You might be wondering what qualifies me to write such a book. Well, I coached the most stubborn person I can think of and turned him into a happier and healthier version of himself. That person is me. I tried different therapies but found them to be only partially effective, or not aligned with my needs. But I never gave up.

I believed that solutions to my problems existed and I just had to find them, no matter what. This was when I began to look inside myself for my own personal power. Once I realized that

I could live the life I dreamed about, I found the solutions and answers to my problems. What were they? Faith and expectation. My faith grew in not only myself, but also in my creator, and the law of expectation took over based off my faith. I started to expect the good I desired.

One of the important reasons I spent so much effort and time writing this book was that telling my story and sharing it aligned with my purpose, since this book can guide almost anybody to start and keep on their journey.

I believe in everything I recommend because it worked for me. There's no reason it can't work for you, too.

However, keep in mind that living a happy and healthy life was not an overnight event for me—it was a journey. Although my journey was much longer than I expected, by sharing my story I hope that you can learn from my progress and take a more direct route.

Some of my experiences were hard to go through, but I know that now I am in a good place for myself.

I officially got divorced on May 18, 2018, and since then I have chosen to not go out on dates because I have been focused on improving myself—my mental, emotional and spiritual levels— building foundations for better romantic and marital relationships in the future instead of just having negative and superficial ones. I believe that now I am almost there. Early in my marriage, my wife had a baby that died prematurely, and we never had any other children.

I took a complete leave of absence from work in July, 2021 to pursue my passion and purpose. I wanted to share the under- standing and wisdom I gained through all those years by writing this book so that others can benefit from it. I learned that writing a book requires a great deal of energy, focus, and time, but I have really enjoyed the process of writing it.

There are many daily activities that give me joy and pleasure, aside from writing. First of all, I meditate twice every day. I practice Hatha yoga, which I learned by taking classes at a nearby studio. I enjoy reading inspirational books because I feel really good and motivated afterward. I walk in nearby parks and sometimes practice forest bathing. All in all, I am living and enjoying life every day and at the same time I visualize my future goals and dreams.

This might not be where I thought I'd be, but I know it is right where I am supposed to be.

The modalities I discovered for myself will surely work for you as long as you follow them consistently with faith and hope, although it may take some time for you to see results. This book is based on my personal experiences from over 20 years. It took me decades to understand these experiences and figure out how to apply them in my life, but I did it. And now I am excited to share my understanding with you.

Let me show you how I changed my life so you can change yours. But first, we have to go back to the beginning, before I achieved my personal successes.

CHAPTER 1

Coping with Depression

Coping with Depression

In my personal growth journey, I learned that there are three states of being that are important to my perception, my ability to live the kind of life I want, and to be depression-free.

1. State of Happiness

Happiness is a state of mind as well as a habit. We have the freedom to choose happiness. It may seem simple, and it is simple. But simple doesn't mean easy. I used to have fun here and there, but I wasn't happy.

It wasn't easy for me to be happy. I was conditioned genetically and environmentally to be unhappy, partially because I was born to unhappy parents.

My father and my mother were both raised by their stepmothers and real fathers, since their biological mothers died when they were under the age of five. They both were the only children in their families, and luckily neither my father nor mother had stepsiblings. Moreover, their real fathers almost always sided with their stepmothers instead of the kids. They were both unhappy. Their similar, unhappy upbringings allowed them to bond over common ground and formed the basis of their relationship.

The main difference between my mother and father was that my father had a temper while my mother didn't. My mother wanted to go to picnics and have fun, while my father wasn't interested in any such things. My mother didn't have an education, and therefore couldn't be financially independent, which is partly why my parents' marriage survived.

She had nowhere else to go and no means of taking care of herself. That kind of marriage isn't set up for happiness. Let me share a story about how my father made us suffer, including himself, although he didn't do it on purpose. This story shows clearly that no matter how much you love your family or children, if you have distorted thinking and conditioning, you will cause your loved ones to suffer. Although good intention is important, it is not enough.

My family decided to go to a picnic on the beach in August of 1990. We bought snacks, prepared meals, and even rented a beach hut. We left around 9 a.m. in the morning and got to the beach (Paradise Point) at 10 a.m. My siblings and I (three brothers, three sisters) played in the waves and rested in the comfort of the hut on and off. We were having a great time. Me, especially, since I really loved the ocean.

Around 4 p.m., while we were having snacks, my father started criticizing us kids, saying that we had bad habits. He began to criticize our studying habits, comparing our grades to the neighbors' kids, and putting us down for not performing as well as them academically.

Since we were trying to have a fun, family outing, it didn't seem like the right time to me for him to bring that up. I reacted defensively and got loud and angry. Very quickly, our good time became a bitter argument, and we all went home unhappy.

With my parents' relationship as an example and the way my father criticized us, I believed it took something artificial to be happy, such as having a certain toy in childhood or having a high-paying job.

I still remember being excited and having fun after getting a toy that I really wanted in 1984, when I was just about 14 years old. It was a two-foot-long candle-powered boat that ran in the water when the wax candle was burning. I played with the boat in the water for many days. At the time, it felt like the boat was the source of my happiness, but I lost interest in the toy after a few weeks. I didn't understand the importance of this experience until 2019, when I realized it wasn't a material object that could make me happy.

Now, in my adulthood, I have gone from not being happy to being happy much more often. Am I happy all the time? No, I am not happy all the time. Nobody is, and that is important to accept on your own journey. If we were happy all the time, we wouldn't know it. We have to experience unhappiness occasionally to know what happiness really is.

2. State of Health

From about 1983 to 2014, from my adolescence and into adulthood, I experienced chronic and recurring health problems. I gained weight during periods of depression. I suffered from a cough for about seven months out of the year. Doctors said the cough was caused by an allergy and suggested I take medication.

But they never knew the root cause. I suffered from constipation, and my doctors believed it to be the result of irritable bowel syndrome (IBS). But they didn't know the root cause of the problem. I used to have an overactive bladder, often waking up three times a night to use the bathroom. There were so many times I couldn't go back to sleep.

I now believe I was not able to digest whatever I used to eat and drink because of my negative mindset. Negative emotions such as anger, resentment, jealousy, envy, bitterness, and fear wreaked havoc on my body, spirit, and mind. The physical body is the instrument of the mind, and as such the body reflects what goes on in the mind. Negative emotions can make the body physically ill, and a troubled spirit can do the same. There are no accidents in life. Everything happens for a reason, according to the natural laws of the universe.

It wasn't until I made huge strides in my personal growth journey that these health issues really started to show improvement, in March of 2021.

My negative mindset had me living in a constant state of stress—both a mental and emotional strain that that can be the result of adverse internal or external circumstances. Stress can be the result of something you experience, such as difficulties at work or in your relationship, or it can be something you create for yourself by always thinking negatively.

Stress affects the physical body by disrupting the respiratory, musculoskeletal, gastrointestinal, reproductive, nervous, cardiovascular, and endocrine systems. It is one of the most common examples of how mental and emotional states can hurt the physical body.

Mental and emotional stress leads to tension in the muscles as the body's natural defense against pain and injury. Chronic muscle tension can cause headaches, migraines, and other musculo-skeletal issues like chronic muscle or joint pain and poor posture, which, in turn, can cause serious bodily injury.

Stress can actually tighten the passageway between the nose and lungs. This causes problems in the respiratory system, like coughing and shortness of breath.

The gut is part of the gastrointestinal system and it is in constant communication with the brain, containing millions of neurons. Stress can actually disrupt the brain-gut communication, leading to all kinds of gastrointestinal discomfort. The millions of bacteria that live in the gut can trigger problems in the brain as a result of stress, such as clear thinking and even triggering emotions.[1]

It's easy to see how my negative mindset and emotional stress was directly causing me to have chronic health issues. It wasn't until I was able to identify the root of the problem that I was able to improve my health. Doctors and medicine could only do so much when they were treating me for allergies and my other chronic physical symptoms, instead of stress. They were focused on my symptoms, not on what was causing them.

Now I am healthier than I ever was, even in my younger years. I don't suffer from constipation and IBS anymore. I am healed from my chronic cough. Am I perfectly healthy? No, but I am much better off. I attribute my health primarily to two factors: adding healthy foods into my life, and more importantly, managing my feelings, thoughts, and behaviors by improving my level of awareness.

3. State of Wealth

I spent a good part of my life pursuing financial wealth only to discover that financial wealth wasn't real wealth. Real wealth comes from happiness and health. However, financial wealth can be a contributing factor to happiness.

Some of the physical health issues I was having were linked to my being stressed about finances and being able to support me and my wife. Ironically, needing more income, as stressful as it was, was also where I began my personal growth journey.

Although money itself and material objects can't create happiness, wealth does play a role. If you are constantly stressed about money, it is really hard to keep yourself happy and healthy.

Part of leading a happy and healthy life is having the wealth to support your existence. That doesn't mean you have to pursue millions of dollars. Just having the money to pay your bills, put food on the table, keep a roof over your head, and have a little fun now and then—like taking that vacation in Italy and supporting your desired lifestyle—is wealth enough!

Wealth is also important because when you are able to improve one aspect of your life, or make it comfortable, it becomes easier to improve other areas of your life. It relieves stress and gives you the confidence to make improvements elsewhere. Another important safety net that financial wealth provides is in giving you the means and security to take care of your physical, mental, emotional, and spiritual health—some therapies, modalities, and treatments can get expensive.

For me, I was able to double my hourly income and cut back on my working hours by about half. I was still financially comfortable and it gave me the time to pursue my personal growth and passions.

So, you see, happiness, health, and wealth are all interconnected and important to living your best life.

Unfortunately, I had to hit rock bottom before I could accept the truth of these three states.

I Was Resentful, Angry, and Depressed_

I started seeing Dr. Nauman Ejaz in 1996 regarding an overactive bladder. He was a practicing urologist in the city of Westland, Michigan.

I was desperate to see him because I would wake up to use the bathroom several times in the middle of the night. On the surface, nighttime urination might not seem like that big of a deal, but it takes away the joy of the most important part of human life – sleep. I felt awful every morning because I could not get a good night's rest.

Unfortunately, I didn't have medical insurance and paid the first office visit with my credit card. I didn't expect to have to deal with long-term treatment. Dr. Ejaz discovered I was a student and didn't have the means to pay for long-term treatment, and when he did, he immediately waived all fees and treated me for more than a year. I am very grateful to him for that. Unknowingly, his kindness and actions became part of my support system.

I was not aware at the time that the harmful emotions of bitterness, resentment, and anger I persistently experienced were taking their toll on my body—that my overactive (stressed out) bladder was just one of the symptoms. I had so many thoughts coming and going so quickly, and my mind was so tired, I couldn't focus on anything.

Dr. Ejaz quickly recognized I was suffering from depression. This is another reason he became such an important source of support in my life. Not a lot of specialists can easily recognize symptoms outside their field of specialty. Without him, I never would have been set on the right path. To him, it was obvious from the way I carried myself and behaved. He suggested that I have a consultation with his psychiatrist friend. But I reacted fiercely. I would not see a psychiatrist no matter what.

First, I didn't think I had any mental disease. I thought that all I needed was "success." To me, success meant a high-paying job, a red Mustang convertible, and nice clothes. Second, I thought he wanted me to change myself and become the kind of moral person my father wanted me to be. I had rebelled against my father's values and whatever he stood for since I was young.

I didn't get along with my father for many reasons. He had a temper and mood swings. He usually communicated angrily. He used to criticize me and my other siblings and put us down by comparing us negatively with other people's kids. He favored my younger sister because she was submissive. She became a doctor only because that's what my father wanted. I was the only rebellious child.

Another reason I rebelled against my father was because of his strict beliefs. There is religiosity (organized religion) and then there is spirituality. He was more religious than spiritual, and he still is. I assumed that Dr. Ejaz wanted me to be religious, and that was why he wanted me to pursue treatments for mental health.

I was wrong. Dr. Ejaz treated me free of charge for more than a year, even though I didn't follow all of his advice. Because of that, I have great respect for him. I don't know why I changed my mind, but I decided to follow his advice after my second visit, which came 60 days later. When I informed him that I was willing to move forward with his advice, he gave me the contact information for a friend of his who was a psychiatrist named Dr. Zakir Khan.

According to Debra Fulgham Bruce, an editorial consultant for WebMD, "about half the people who have depression never get it diagnosed or treated."[2] Having depression is different from being sad. Feeling sad, lonely, or depressed is "a normal reaction to life's struggles," but when these feelings become "overwhelming, cause physical symptoms, and last for long periods of time," you need to see a doctor.[3]

I went to see Dr. Khan and explained to him in detail my symptoms and problems. He prescribed me Effexor, an antidepressant. He also felt that I needed psychotherapy, but he didn't have the time to offer it to me. He knew I wasn't insured and didn't refer me to any other psychotherapists who would require insurance or payments I couldn't afford. Therefore, I didn't receive any kind of psychotherapy.

I took Effexor once a day for a couple months, but I only noticed minor relief. I went to see Dr. Khan again and informed him about my condition. As a result, he increased my dosage to twice a day. I started to feel pleasure from time to time, but I was getting triggered even more often by circumstances and events. I called him 35 days after taking his new recommended dose and explained over the phone how I was doing.

He finally increased my dosage to three times a day. I became slow to respond to even simple things, like somebody asking me for directions. I felt like my mind was getting somewhat numb. I thought three times a day was too much for me. I didn't feel like calling him again, since I wasn't satisfied with the results I had received so far.

However, I am still grateful to him for providing me completely free treatment. Though my experience with medication wasn't satisfactory, the mental health care system has changed a lot since the '90s. There are a lot more medications available now, and it is common practice these days to try different kinds, or even a different mix of medications, until good, steady, progress is seen.

Unfortunately, I wasn't knowledgeable about other medications and couldn't ask for a change. Even if I had been, the dose of medication I was on had altered my behaviors and thoughts so much that I wasn't in a mindset to make such a suggestion.

Depression is different from having other physical illnesses or injuries, such as a broken leg, because people can't see your depression nor can they sympathize with you because everyone's experience is so personal.

Although shoulder pain can't be seen with the naked eye either, the individual with shoulder pain usually consults a physician or physical therapist because shoulder pain is uncomfortable to tolerate. Trained professionals can feel stiffness in the joint, test range of motion, and visibly determine if the shoulder is moving the way it is supposed to. But in many cases, people don't even know they are suffering from depression or how they could get treatment.

I Made the Wrong Decision

Have you ever made a decision that you regretted over and over again but realized after many years that it had to be made so that you could learn the lesson you needed to learn? Well, I did, and I would never forget the lesson I learned.

I decided to pursue my BBA in computer information systems (CIS) in 1997, since I only had 55 credit hours left to finish my degree. I thought I would finish my degree easily in a year, but depression had a different plan. I didn't yet know I wouldn't be able to achieve anything because I was too busy fighting off depression, but I'd soon learn this.

I flunked both fall 1997 and winter 1998 semesters, since I wasn't able to focus and study my course material as well as I needed. I wasn't able to think properly due to numbness of my mind. My sense of failure exacerbated my depression. I started focusing on my utter failure in both semesters. I felt like it was the end of the world. I lost whatever confidence I had. I didn't know what to do. Moreover, I had accumulated student loan debt.

I Found "Hope" in November 1998

I found hope in November 1998 when an acquaintance of mine stopped by my apartment. I was not answering his phone calls and he was concerned about me. I didn't bother answering phone calls because I didn't care much about anything. He had recently started an IT job after completing his BBA in CIS.

We had both been pursuing degrees in CIS, which is how I came to know him. He suggested that I could still get an IT job in Windows networking by doing Microsoft certified systems engineer (MCSE) certification. He said, "You could still get a job based on MCSE certifications and finish your degree on a part-time basis while doing your job."

I really liked his idea. I somehow became hopeful and excited again. I started searching for a decent IT institute, and found one in the city of Southfield, MI called Computech.

I started my MCSE training in January of 1999. I paid the $10,000 in tuition fees through credit cards, since I thought I could easily pay off the balance after getting a job within six to eight months. Moreover, I didn't want to go through the hassle of applying for student loans. Well, I was dead wrong. Yes, I got my MCSE certifications in six months, in June 1999, but getting a job became a nightmare. I worked hard not only to get the MCSE certification, but also getting basic hands-on experience while getting certified.

I had my résumé put together by a professional résumé service. I invested in a nice navy blue suit that looked good on me. I asked a few acquaintances that had IT jobs to help me get a job in their companies. I applied for a lot of entry-level positions online as well as in person. I followed up assertively and politely after applying for each job. I did everything I possibly could. I even passed the first interviews on a couple occasions—a lot of IT jobs have a two to three interview process. But in the end, I didn't get any job offers after searching for a year and a half.

Depression Turned into Severe Depression

I gave up the hope of actually having an IT job in November 2000. The sense of failure multiplied many times over to the point that I considered myself to be a failure instead of seeing the reality that I just failed to achieve my goals. I acquired cognitive distortions and thinking on all of these distortions:

1. I failed to achieve my bachelor's degree, and that made me a loser.

2. I failed to get an IT job, so I must be a loser.

3. I accumulated huge credit card and student loan debt. I was very uncomfortable with my debt. I was concerned with how I was going to pay it back without having a decent job.

4. Other people I knew got IT jobs, so I thought I was the only unlucky one. This wasn't actually true, since I did know other people who didn't get jobs in IT either. But nonetheless, I became jealous and resentful.

5. I started perceiving myself as a victim, and I acquired a victim mindset. I thought that I worked really hard but I was actually denied success.

6. I started cursing the divine (God).

7. I lost all the hope and expectation that makes life worth living.

8. I wasn't able to focus on anything positive in my life.

9. I was only able to work on a part-time basis due to the worst physical and mental state I'd ever experienced. All these distorted thought patterns exacerbated my depression to severe depression.

Deeper Emotional Issues

I believe having depression was a way for my body to tell me that something was not right, although I was not aware of it at the time. I became aware of those deeper emotional issues within me once I gained some level of awareness in November 2019.

From 2000 to 2014, I was having a miserable and painful existence with my emotional, mental, spiritual, and physical health. I was lost, floundering, and couldn't make sense of my own existence. I thought that was my fate and there was nothing I could do about it.

However, things began to turn around in 2014. I joined an XSport gym and started doing workouts with a personal trainer that January. Movement and exercise are so important to mental health, especially with the production of endorphins.

I enrolled in a 13-month online personal-growth coaching program in June 2015, and that is how I started my journey.

By 2019, I started becoming more aware of myself. I had been trying to achieve outward symbols of success such as a high-paying

IT job and bachelor's degree to hide and mask my low self-esteem, lack of confidence, and lack of self-love.

Even if I had been successful in school and my career, I would not have found inner peace and happiness, but I didn't realize that until much later.

You might be wondering, "Why didn't you have self-esteem, confidence, and self-love?" Well, I went through many emotional and physical traumas in my life. I got bullied and attacked in school, my parents criticized me and my other siblings consistently, and I was physically tortured and humiliated.

Let me share one incident from 1984, when I was 15 years old. I was in the ninth grade and another classmate beat me up on the school premises. When Moin came to fight with me, for no reason, I was both angry and fearful at the same time. It is interesting that we human beings can feel more than one emotion at the same time. As usual, I had more fear than anger at the time of the incident and I let Moin beat me up.

I lost respect for myself, thinking I was a coward for a long time. We human beings don't have much control over how we get conditioned, both genetically and environmentally, from the time of conception in the mother's womb to the time we grow up. That doesn't mean we can't overcome that conditioning with self-awareness. I have more confidence now because I accepted that I'm not a coward.

It is a simple formula to determine whether we fight or give in:

Anger -> Fear = We Fight

Fear -> Anger = We Succumb

Drug Therapy/Pharmacotherapy

Hopelessness and depression turned to severe depression. I had suicidal thoughts from January 2001 until May 2002. I was thinking about how to end my life without going through pain. I wanted to get my hands on a certain drug, because it seemed to be a painless way to end my life.

I didn't want to be alive, but fear stopped me from taking action to end my life. The fear of surviving the attempt seemed even more dreadful. I was restless and anxious during this period. I was driving a taxi a couple days a week—I wasn't capable of working full-time, anyway. I didn't know what the hell I was doing.

I was in such bad shape that anybody could see I was suffering. I didn't feel like seeing people I knew because I was ashamed of myself. An acquaintance of mine came to see me and found me in this awful condition. Out of sympathy, he provided me with the contact information for another psychiatrist in February of 2001. Initially, I didn't feel like seeing another psychiatrist due to the bad experience I had with the previous one. But somehow I went to see Dr. Rizwan Shah.

He was happy to provide me with proper treatment free of charge. The keywords here are "proper" and "free." Dr. Shah was willing to see me once or twice a week at his residence depending on my needs. I felt supported beyond simply getting handed a prescription.

He prescribed me many medicines, and he changed them if one wasn't helping me. I tried Depakote, Risperdal, Zoloft, Paxil, Abilify, Lithium, and Xanax. No matter which one of these medicines I tried, I was having a hard time dealing with one side effect or another such as insomnia, drowsiness, nervousness, nausea, constipation, diarrhea, or dry mouth. It seemed like every medicine I tried came with negative side effects.

I took different medicines for a year and half consistently. After that year and a half, I started taking only Xanax, and only when I felt I really needed it, for the next six months. Although I was not healed or cured, drug therapy helped me during the period I was dealing with suicidal thoughts.

It was like a bandage on my most severe wounds, allowing me to move forward.

Lessons Learned

Drug therapy can be an effective treatment for depression,[4] but it's also important to consider combining that treatment with some type of talk therapy, depending on your needs. Keep two things in mind with regard to drug therapy. First, you have to deal with side effects, and sometimes they can be challenging.[5] Second, drug therapy doesn't cure depression, it manages the symptoms.[6] To truly heal, you need to invest money, time, and effort to look within for real causes, not just symptoms. In my experience, depression is something that is very important to deal with holistically.

Filing for Bankruptcy in 2002

I had debt on four different credit cards, and I struggled to make payments on time since they all had different due dates—which was made even more difficult when I was dealing with severe depression. I wasn't able to focus on anything, so on multiple occasions I missed making payments on time. Therefore, the credit card companies raised the interest rates. I spoke with them and tried to reach an understanding. I explained to them my situation, but they didn't want to lower the interest rates. I kept making minimum payments, but the principal credit card balance stayed almost the same.

I discussed this situation with my informal mentor, Dr. Ejaz. He suggested that I file for bankruptcy. It was not an easy decision for me, but after thinking about it long and hard, I agreed. I hired an attorney and filed for bankruptcy. My credit history and credit score got screwed up and I wasn't able to get any credit card for a long time. I had to rebuild my credit card history from the ground up.

I Received Counseling

My new psychiatrist recommended I get therapy to deal with my cognitive distortions. I didn't have insurance that covered therapy, so I did what I could to find affordable options. I found such an option at Eastern Michigan University. The psychology department offered counseling and therapy from students who were doing their PhDs with the intention of becoming psychotherapists. Hour-long sessions cost only $15, and that was the best option for me at the time.

The way counseling works is that you talk about and work through your personal problems. The counselor helps you address your problems in a positive way by helping you to clarify the issues, explore options, develop strategies, and increase self-awareness. Counseling can help relieve distress, build resilience,[7] and improve self-esteem.[8]

I started receiving counseling in August 2001, and it continued on for roughly 55 weeks. My first counselor was a student who ultimately didn't have the experience I needed for my treatment, and I wasn't yet ready to receive healing. I was blaming everybody and anybody for what I was going through—God, my parents, my luck, my circumstances.

I didn't receive any lasting and long-term benefits, though I received short-term benefits. I used to feel lighter and better by expressing my feelings. The counselor listened to me and we explored my options. However, counseling can be an effective modality depending on your needs and the expertise of your counselor. You have to be ready to receive healing.

It wasn't until 2007 that I found a therapy that was more effective for me, which is discussed in detail in Chapter 3.

Psychotherapy

There are many psychotherapeutic practices out there. Some common types are:

- Counseling

- Cognitive behavioral therapy

- Hypnosis (hypnotherapy)

- Eye movement desensitization and reprocessing (EMDR therapy)[9]

My Tips About Finding the Right Psychotherapist

- Read my description about different types of psychotherapies offered below and ask yourself what kind of therapy you really need.

- Do online research about the psychotherapists you are considering.

- Discuss the healing goals you would like to accomplish with your therapist.

- You can read reviews online and look at work experience and education of the therapist, along with other factors.

Different Types of Psychotherapy

1. COGNITIVE BEHAVIOR THERAPY

Cognitive behavior therapy (CBT) works on the idea that "how we think (cognition), how we feel (emotion), and how we act (behavior), all interact together."[10] Therefore, CBT aims to help you identify and challenge unhelpful thoughts and behaviors and to learn practical self-help strategies.

2. HYPNOTHERAPY/HYPNOSIS

Hypnotherapy "uses guided relaxation, intense concentration, and focused attention to achieve a heightened state of awareness that is sometimes called a trance."[11] The person's attention is so focused while in this state that anything going on around them is "temporally blocked out or ignored. In this naturally-occurring state ... the person may focus his or her attention on specific thoughts or task."[12]

Hypnotherapy can be effective because it accesses the subconscious mind, where traumas and deeper issues reside. Hypnotherapists might enable people to perceive some things differently, such as blocking the awareness of pain.

A couple of things to consider when looking into hypnotherapy as an option:

*It is not yet recognized to be an effective modality by insurance companies, and won't be covered by insurance.

*There are many ways hypnotherapy is practiced, so you have to do your own research about what type of hypnotherapy you need. You can inquire about the certifications and credentials hypnotherapists possess.[13]

3. EYE MOVEMENT DESENSITIZATION AND REPROCESSING THERAPY (EMDR)

EMDR therapy "does not require talking in detail about the distressing issue, or homework between sessions. EMDR, rather than focusing on changing the emotions, thoughts, or behaviors resulting from the distressing issue, allows the brain to resume its natural healing process."[14] EMDR is designed to resolve unprocessed traumatic memories in the brain.

The Most important Lesson Is the Importance of Hope

When I first began pursuing therapy options at Eastern Michigan University, I wasn't ready to heal. I wasn't truly ready to face myself and my traumas and work through them. I was aware enough that I knew something was wrong and something needed to change, but I wasn't ready to commit to what I had to do to make those changes. That was because I still hadn't rediscovered hope.

While it is important to find the right kind of therapy that works for you and your needs, it will only be effective if you are truly ready to heal—if you are hopeful for your future.

I was motivated, ambitious, and working hard on three different occasions. First, when I was pursuing my bachelor's degree, when I was doing my MCSE certification, and when I was looking for a job. This was because I had a goal to work toward and, more importantly, I had hope and expectations.

The most important fact is that as long as you have hope you can face almost any challenge. I can eat shitty food and live in a shitty apartment as long as I have something to look forward to. But I had false hope based on my five physical senses: seeing, hearing, smelling, tasting, and touching. The true and real hope can only come if you have awareness—the awareness of who you are and what you are capable of. We are spiritual beings living in physical bodies and possess intellect. We can achieve anything we truly desire within the bounds of reason. I was missing true hope, so I did not believe that

CHAPTER 2

The Post-Depression Period

The Post-Depression Period

I **started** living my life in the fall of 2004, when I came out of my long depression cycle. I started to think of possibilities. It feels like yesterday. I was happy coming out of my depression, though keep in mind that it is not the same happiness you experience when you become peaceful inside after being transformed. It is a unique kind of happiness felt by an individual who comes out of depression and being happy that he is not depressed anymore.

I also knew that any relatively big negative event or circumstance could easily trigger me back into the dark world of depression, so I had fear inside of me. I had many dreadful "what if" scenarios troubling me.

I was living in Ypsilanti, Michigan and eager to enjoy the fall season, as it is my favorite season. It is great to see, hear, and smell fall, especially the smells. I love the way fall smells, especially when I stroll around beautiful local lakes in the evening—my desires for love, intimacy, sex, and delicious food multiply a thousand times. I have trouble describing these feelings in words. I wish that time would stop and I could live in that feeling forever. I started to have fun here and there. I would go to The Edge Bar a couple nights a week, eat delicious, spicy food at restaurants, and, of course, take strolls around the lake and enjoy the fall.

Don't be deceived, I still had anger, bitterness, a sense of failure, and a victim mindset within me, it is just that all those feelings went down from my conscious mind to my subconscious mind. For the time being, I started to focus more on the beauty of women than the idea of how unlucky I was.

I Was Having Fun Then but See Now That I Wasn't Happy

It wasn't until later that I discovered that there is a huge difference between being happy and having fun. Fun is a momentary and surface feeling we experience when we enjoy delicious food or have good sex. Fun has more to do with our five senses.

Happiness Is a State of Mind and a Way of Being

You don't need a specific reason to be happy, but you do have to cultivate the state of happiness unless you were born with it. I was not born happy, since I was born to unhappy parents. I recall very few occasions when I saw my parents laugh, let alone be happy. I don't think I heard a joke in our home, especially when I was a child. Happiness was not on the menu of the things they wanted.

Neither of my parents knew how to communicate assertively. My father had a bad temper and used to easily get angry and loud. On the other hand, my mother was passive. I was affected by my parent's behaviors. I would sometimes behave passive aggressively, while other times I would behave outright aggressively. Although I acquired a sense of humor in my mid-20s, it was a crude sense of humor.

Happiness is the lasting and deep feeling that we experience when we wake up rejuvenated and happy after a deep and restful sleep or go to bed happy eagerly awaiting life tomorrow.

Happiness can be found in the most unexpected places. For instance, the 1955 movie *To Catch a Thief* makes me happy. It lifts me out of sadness every time I watch it. I have watched it at least 11 times, mostly when I was feeling unhappy. It transports me to post-World War II French Riviera where life is happening at a slow pace and offering finer things.

I can never forget the scenes in which the gorgeous Grace Kelly and handsome Cary Grant are watching awesome fireworks over the water from the window of a luxurious hotel suite or when she takes him for a joy ride in her classic 1953 Sunbeam Alpine Mk I, passing beautiful scenery and eventually enjoying a picnic in the woods where they were invisible but could see the Riviera.

You might be wondering how watching a movie could possibly make me happy. Well, you have to use your imagination to grasp the concept. Suppose you have two best friends, one of whom is a movie director and the other is a producer, and they agree to make a movie based on your dream life. Use your imagination. How would you feel when you watch this movie based on your dream life? Cary Grant is living parts of my dream life in *To Catch a Thief.* When I watch it, I feel inspired, motivated, and uplifted. It is more than the fleeting happiness I'd get from just watching a movie I enjoy.

Have you ever noticed that strong desires make you want to do things you normally wouldn't consider doing? Well, that is how it was for me. I did whatever I could to fulfill my desires.

You see, the burning desire was inside of me. It was the essence of who I was. The desire to live life where I could enjoy beauty in all shapes and forms, the beauty of women, the beauty of the environment, and the beauty of clothing. I was hoping to meet someone who would guide me and maybe even mentor me to move toward the life I longed for.

Guidance Into Hope and Possibility

Happiness is a habit and a state of mind. However, life is dynamic, not static, meaning we have to keep moving toward our vision and dream life. As such, we all need people and mentors who can guide us so that we can start moving toward that path. It is also true that we humans tend to gravitate toward people who help us in any way, shape, or form. You might be wondering, how do we find such people?

Life is strange, and as such we find people and things we hope to bring into our lives in places we are not really expecting at all. I found guidance in hope and possibility at the place I was not expecting.

In January 1999, I met such a guiding man by mere accident. Vijay Kumar and I were both being trained for MCSE at the IT institute Computech in Southfield, MI.

He had a high-paying IT job and was getting his MCSE certification just to enhance his credentials, as he already had eight years work experience in his field. I, on the other hand, was getting an MCSE certification so I could get an entry-level position. At the time, he was 56 years old and I was 36. I am showing the age difference to show the kind of relationship we had. It wasn't a friendship among equals, but sort of an informal mentorship.

It was somewhere in the month of January when we were introduced to each other. He helped me figure out a computer networking issue that had stumped me in the institute's lab. From this incident onward he started teaching me about Microsoft Windows networking, either before the class started or at the end of class.

Vijay and I exchanged contact information and stayed in touch with each other. He did the best he could to help me get a networking job. He provided me some job leads and helped me get interviews. I would go see him from time to time even after I gave up looking for a job. He offered me many ideas to move forward, toward living the life I dreamed about, such as renting a kiosk in the mall and selling niche products. But there was one particular idea he offered that changed my life completely.

I Really Liked the Idea

In September of 2004, Vijay invited me to come see him in the beautiful mall located in Southfield, MI. He had just returned from his visit to the Virginia and Washington, D.C. area. He mentioned to me that he personally knew people in the area who were making $80,000 to $100,000 a year working as appliance repair subcontractors.

Furthermore, he said he could help me start working with those subcontractors if I would be willing to get some experience in the appliance repair field and move to Virginia. I was so excited. My heart rate elevated, my palms got sweaty, and I had butterflies in my stomach. In my imagination, I was already living my dream life—enjoying the company of beautiful girls, eating delicious, spicy food at fancy restaurants, wearing nice clothes, and driving my red Mustang convertible.

My Thought Pattern and Way of Being

I got motivated and excited again after seeing an opportunity to achieve my dream life. There were two things to observe mindfully. First, the concept of my dream life stayed the same. The only thing that changed for me was how to go about achieving it. In the period between 1997 and 2000, I thought the way to achieve this was by getting an IT job. Now it was through being an appliance repair subcontractor in the Virginia and Washington, D.C. area.

The second thing to observe about me was that I can stay motivated and enthusiastic as long as I can see the opportunity through my five senses.

Lessons need to be learned, and although I had been through so much suffering and so many challenges, I didn't grow to be a higher and better person. I had been living a materialistic, shallow life.

My Plan to Work Toward My Dream Life

- My goal was to start working as an appliance repair contractor in the Virginia and Washington, D.C. area and to make $80,000 to $100,000 a year.

- The must-have for me was to acquire working experience of repairing appliances.

- The only way I could get experience was to get a job as a repair technician at any appliance repair company.

- That was a challenge because appliance repair companies usually give a job to candidates who already have working experience or possess some kind of technical certification. The solution to this challenge was getting a certification from a good technical institute.

Northwestern Technological Institute

I started searching for technical institutes and I found Northwestern Technological Institute (NWTI), which looked decent. They offered an eight-month appliance repair theory and a hands-on training certification program. The total cost was going to be $10,000.

Paying for the certification was a challenge. Not only did I not have any savings whatsoever, I had debt from student loans I accumulated while I was doing my bachelor degree in computer information systems.

I was afraid of getting more student loan debt due to my past experience of going to school and then not getting a job. I thought about this challenge day and night. An employment agency I was in contact with was willing to pay the tuition only if I chose to go to community college, because they had a limited budget and they had to divide their funds fairly among many candidates.

I arranged a meeting with the manager of the employment agency and spoke to him in person. I looked in his eyes and said that I understand that paying a total of $10,000 toward a single candidate's certification was way beyond their limit, but I would make good use of it. It would not only help me but also help the community and industry.

I believed he saw something in me and he unexpectedly approved the funds I needed to attend Northwestern Technological Institute. I am truly grateful to him and the taxpayers.

In January 2006, I started doing appliance repair and HVAC certification at NWTI. I was excited and motivated to be moving forward, but I still had a negative thought pattern. I was dwelling on my past failures. Failure can cause severe damage to a person's self-esteem and confidence. I was comparing myself with others in such a way that I found myself to be unlucky and a victim. I had a hard time focusing on my course material. I was also having mild depression, but I wanted to avoid taking medicine if I could.

I talked with Vijay about how to best deal with mild depression and having a hard time focusing on course material. He suggested trying quality herbal and dietary supplements instead of prescription drugs, since he knew I was sensitive to side effects from prescription medicine. Moreover, he said if I didn't see any noticeable results within 40 days, I could always go back to the drug therapy route.

My Introduction to Herbal and Dietary Supplements

In 2006, there weren't as many online companies selling dietary and herbal supplements and products, at least not that I was aware of. I searched locally in the yellow pages and found Ancient Formula in the city of Ann Arbor.

I went to Ancient Formula and met with Jack, the man at the cash register, who was an herbalist and the owner of the shop. I explained to him my problems of mild depression, negative thought patterns, lack of energy on some days, and inability to focus.

Jack was damn good in the field of herbal and dietary supplements. He provided me two supplements, the names of which now escape me, but they were intended to help me focus so that I could study my course material as well as calm my body and mind to produce feelings of joy instead of feeling depressed. He also prepared a customized formula for me, which I picked up the next week.

Those products and formulas calmed my body and mind and I started to feel better. I was able to focus on my course material and studies. I had more energy to do things. The symptoms of mild depression went away.

Jack and I became close and I started hanging out at his shop on some evenings where other individuals also used to hang out. We would occasionally drink wine and discuss various topics such as culture, cuisine, politics, the European way of life, and herbs.

Certified!

The herbal and dietary supplements helped me stay focused and positive. I studied hard and participated in the hands-on training labs. I was the first person to arrive at class and last one to leave, asking questions of my instructors. I never missed any classes or hands-on labs. The journey of getting my certification started in January 2006 and ended when I graduated on August 23, 2006.

I had been using dietary and herbal supplements since February 2005 to successfully treat many conditions, such as frequent nighttime urination (overactive bladder), allergies, IBS, severe cough, cold, flu and occasional sleep issues.

As far as my experience of healing is concerned, some conditions got healed for good, but some needed to be managed with a continuous use of herbal supplements. The thing I like about this form of therapy is they usually have no side effects—at least I didn't experience any.

S-Adenosyl-L-methionine (SAMe) is a naturally occurring molecule in the human body that influences chemicals involved in the brain chemistry related to depression and other disorders like osteoarthritis and chronic liver conditions.

David Mischoulon, a professor of psychiatry at Harvard, has postulated that SAMe, St. John's Wort, and fish oil capsules containing omega-3 are effective in treating depression.[15]

Though herbal supplements are easier to come by than prescription medications, it is still important to seek professional help in regard to proper dosing, quality of the product, reputable places to purchase products, instructions for proper and safe use, the right supplement for your symptoms, and long-term care. Mischoulon reminds us, "One of the main things I emphasize to patients is that they should not self-medicate with any of these supplements, especially if they are already taking other medications."[16]

Dietary and Herbal Supplements

Let me first explain what exactly dietary supplements are. Dietary supplements are manufactured products in the form of pills, capsules, tablets, powders, and liquids. As the name suggests, dietary supplements are not replacements, but are intended to supplement an individual's diet to provide certain physical or even mental benefits.

Take Methylsulfonylmethane (MSM), for example. It is a compound with anti-inflammatory benefits. MSM is sold as a dietary supplement and it interacts with the body by suppressing the immune system receptors that activate an inflammatory response in the body. Inflammation is a natural immune response to injury, but sometimes can become a chronic and very painful condition. MSM can help alleviate those conditions.[17]

Herbal supplements are a type of dietary supplement containing one or more herbs, sometimes called botanicals.[18] Dietary and herbal supplements can and do alleviate diseases and conditions by nourishing the body. There are many factors that determine how beneficial dietary and herbal supplements can be with regard to alleviating symptoms of disease:

- The quality of dietary supplements is very important. One way to ensure you are buying quality products is by doing research about the company that makes the product. Look at how the company started, what the company philosophy is, how long the company has been in existence, and, most importantly, if the company has a physical street address. There are so many online private labelers selling products under the disguise of companies, but they are middlemen selling synthetic supplements, vitamins, and minerals. Please note: Dietary and herbal supplements are not regulated by the FDA.

- I try to buy supplements in liquid form if possible since the body can digest liquid much more easily than capsules and pills. I can also mix liquid into tea, which makes drinking it part of my normal daily routine.

- Supplements needs to be taken consistently for a period of one to nine weeks in order to see some noticeable results.

- You need to find the supplements right for your condition and symptoms, and if you don't know how to find them, you should seek professional help.

- Supplements may or may not work depending on the nature of the conditions. It also depends how severe and chronic the condition is. For instance, supplements helped me with mild depression, but they wouldn't be helpful in severe depression.

- Taking supplements are much more effective if an individual also works with the mind to improve their beliefs and paradigms.

- I had no understanding whatsoever when I started using dietary and herbal supplements. I experienced healing, though symptoms came back in periods of high stress circumstances. I still believe taking quality dietary and herbal supplements is a good strategy as individuals get relief with no side effects.

I Only Use Whole Food-Based Supplements

I believe in consuming whole food-based supplements, and as such I never purchase or consume synthetic supplements, vitamins, or minerals. In my opinion, they can cause harm to the body and mind instead of providing benefits. Therefore, it makes no sense wasting money on cheap synthetic products that the human body can't absorb and digest. It is your responsibility as the buyer to inquire about and make sure that supplements you are buying are indeed made from whole food plant-based sources.

Natural Nutrients vs. Synthetic Nutrients

NATURAL NUTRIENTS

Natural nutrients are "obtained from whole food sources in the diet."[19] Natural nutrients are the vitamins, minerals, antioxidants, and other compounds we gain through a whole, healthy diet. Therefore, they exist naturally in plants, meats, and other whole, raw food items.

SYNTHETIC NUTRIENTS

Artificial nutrients are made to mimic natural nutrients but are made from chemical sources rather than natural compounds. A lot of the dietary supplements on the market are made synthetically.[20] When looking for supplements that are natural, look at the label or company sources to ensure they are 100 percent plant- or animal-based.[21] Supplements that list ingredients individually, rather than listing a single, 100 percent ingredient, are most likely synthetic.

The production process of synthetic nutrients is very different to the way plants and animals create them. So, despite having a similar structure, your body may react differently to synthetic nutrients. They might not be digested or assimilated into the body properly.[22]

I am going to share some brands and companies that I have used, but I have no relationship with these brands whatsoever. Moreover, I tried only certain products of these brands. I found the products through these companies to be good quality and effective in my needs. They are:

1. New Chapter Perfect Calm (multivitamin and minerals stress formula) to enhance overall mood and combat oxidative stress. This also includes cultural herbal blends to provide immune and digestive support.

2. Irwin Naturals Power to Sleep PM contains melatonin and GABA, which are the keys to maintaining normal sleep cycles. It also contains L-Theanine, which increases alpha brain waves.

3. Nordic Naturals Omega-3 for cognition, heart health, and eye and immune support.

4. Himalaya StressCare supports adrenal function and helps relax and calm your mind and body to lower stress and provide even energy and vitality throughout the day and restful relaxation at night.

CHAPTER 3

Working Toward My Goals and Dreams

Working Toward My Goals and Dreams

I graduated from Northwestern Technological Institute on August 23, 2006 with excitement, hope, and fear. I was hopeful and excited about making $80,000 to $100,000 a year in my near future once I started working as an appliance repair contractor. But due to my past failure, I also had lots of fear and doubt whether I would be able to get hired in my new field.

I searched for entry-level positions in the appliance repair field in a 40-miles radius from where I resided in Michigan. I wasn't getting good responses from employers. I suppose it was because Michigan had a lot of unemployment at the time. The "Big Three"—General Motors, Fiat Chrysler, and Ford—were a big part of the Michigan economy, and they were going through a lot of restructuring at the time.[23]

While it is much easier to make money as an independent subcontractor for appliance repair in a metropolitan area such as the

D.C.-Maryland-Virginia area, it is equally hard to be trained as an entry-level technician there, since this area is a very expensive place to live. There's a lot more competition for lower-paying jobs and a higher cost of living had the potential to put me in more debt.

I wanted to train in entry-level positions in an area where I could afford to live off lower wages before applying for the higher-paying, $80,000 to $100,000 jobs in the greater metropolitan areas.

I applied for a technician's job at Sears, not knowing that the job was actually located in Flagstaff, AZ. I interviewed over the phone and they offered me the job. I accepted right away as this was the first time a job in my field was ever offered to me. I couldn't even think about saying no.

It was the easiest decision, but it was also the hardest. It meant moving all the way to Flagstaff, starting all over in a new part of the country, knowing that eventually I would need to move again to the Virginia and Washington, D.C. area after getting one or two years of job experience.

However, I was not focused on all the hassle involved. The only thing in mind was my dream of making money and living the life I longed to live.

Have you ever completely changed your life in just one week? Well, I did. And I don't recommend it.

Things happened fast. I graduated on August 23 and seven days later I was living in Flagstaff. Before leaving Michigan, I searched online, found a one-bedroom apartment, and wired them a deposit. I made arrangements with my current landlord and he let me leave in a week. I fit everything I possibly could in my car and threw away whatever I couldn't.

By the way, I had a 1985 Toyota Corolla and it was a stick shift. I bought it for $500 and it leaked oil. I had to add oil on a continuous basis. I drove 1,883 miles to Flagstaff in three days, covering roughly 627 miles a day. I passed majestic scenery during my journey, and I wish I had been in the frame of mind to enjoy it.

But I was consumed with fearful thoughts: "What if my car breaks down?" "What if I get there and they change their mind about the job?" "What if the apartment falls through?"

Flagstaff is located at an elevation of 7,000 feet, and due to thinness of air, acute mountain sickness can hit those who visit. I went to see my would-be manager, Greg, the same day I arrived.

Upon arriving, I faced a crisis yet again. Although I had theoretical knowledge and understanding about my chosen field, I had no mechanical aptitude whatsoever.

Put bluntly, I didn't even know how to hold the nut driver or vice grips. I was a book person and I read a lot of books on various topics. I learned to use some tools in my practical labs during my training, but I never really respected people who used them for work—I looked down on people like mechanics, plumbers, and handymen who made a living using tools.

My Manager, Jeff, Saved My Career at His Expense

My manager, Jeff, allocated five weeks for me to be trained, riding along with senior technicians including Ben and David. I was far from ready to go out to customers' residences to repair appliances on my own after receiving a five-week training. Jeff was so disappointed with my performance that he actually vowed to never hire somebody over the phone or out of state. He had to meet his production target for his crew and that was the reason he hired me, assuming I would be an asset.

On the contrary, I was a liability for Sears and Jeff because senior technicians had to spend their time training me. Jeff was faced with a tough choice, as he had to either fire me or give me more training. Although he was very disappointed with my performance, he was impressed with my motivation and attitude.

I have to be fair to Sears and Jeff. Five weeks should have been enough to train someone, provided you have basic mechanical aptitudes, which I clearly lacked, even though I had spent eight months in a certification program.

Jeff said to me, "Since I brought you here from Ypsilanti, Michigan, I am going to provide you much more training."

He ended up providing me with 15 weeks of training and that was something Jeff had not done in his management history at Sears. I had to learn as quickly as possible to be able to survive. If I lost my job with Sears, I would not be able to support myself doing any other job. Most likely, I would go through a depression cycle, and who knows how severe this one would be.

My Mentor and Friend, Ben

Ben started to mentor me in the art and science of the in-home appliance repair industry. I started to see him in his house after work and learn not only how to use tools but also other aspects of the job. I went to see him every day, and yes, I mean every day including weekends. He is and was the best HVAC and appliance repair technician I ever saw. He had a great heart, too.

I am so grateful to Ben for everything he did for me.

David and Lisa Helped Me in Ways They Can't Imagine

I was doing the 15th and last week of my training and was ready to drive my own Sears van to provide in-home appliance services. I was riding with David on that day when I fell in a customer's yard leaving his house. A dog tried to jump on me, and although the dog was on a leash, when I tried to move backward I fell on the ground. I had no medical insurance.

I wasn't in a lot of pain after the fall, but I was scared of the possibility of needing surgery. I had X-rays, I was given a sling to wear for two months, which restricted my mobility. I was able to drive an automatic vehicle with my left hand, though not my own stick shift car. I was mentally and emotionally exhausted because I wanted to get out of Arizona as soon as possible, and this delay was upsetting. It felt like my life stopped going forward, especially since I was new to the area and I didn't know many people there.

David and his wife, Lisa, helped me in so many ways. First, they made efforts to get me covered with worker's compensation, which wasn't easy at all. Second, they helped me find an orthopedic surgeon in Phoenix, almost 182 miles away (about a four-hour drive), since they weren't able to find a surgeon in the vicinity. Third, they took me to the surgeon in Phoenix and brought me back, which meant David had to take a day off. Fourth, I resided with them for almost a month in their house while I healed. Last but not the least, they calmed my mind by giving me hope. I was scared about many things—what would happen if I needed surgery, how long would it take to heal, and when would I be able to go back to work?

I am truly grateful to David and Lisa.

I am truly grateful to the Sears repair crew, especially Jeff, Ben, and David. Without all the help these guys provided me, I would have literally been on the street and possibly fallen back into the dark world of depression and hopelessness.

Nature was constantly teaching me this lesson, but I didn't learn this lesson until many years passed.

Lesson Learned

A great person is not the one with lots of money or a nice car or the highest education, but the person who contributes to being part of the community on a higher level.

In my opinion, one of the most important benefits I received working for Sears was having medical insurance. I can't express how relived I felt knowing I could see doctors and therapists of my choice without getting favors from doctors. I just had to pay a co-pay and I was happy paying that. I got medical insurance after working for Sears for 90 days. I also gained confidence at work after running service calls on my own. After achieving more confidence at work and medical insurance, the first thing I did was start seeing a professional psychotherapist.

Cognitive Behavioral Therapy

I received cognitive behavioral therapy once a week for three months in 2007. My therapist was very experienced and she diagnosed my emotional issues correctly and did the best she could to help me. The therapy had some lasting benefits, though my emotional wounds and mental blocks were far from completely removed.

Cognitive behavioral therapy (CBT) is a type of talk therapy. In a CBT session, a trained counselor talks you through recognizing inaccurate or negative thought patterns so you can have a clearer perspective on situations. This allows you to respond to these situations more effectively.[24]

Healing is a journey, not an event, and as such receiving cognitive behavioral therapy was a good start toward healing.

Nature Had Been Trying to Teach Me a Lesson that I Had Yet to Learn

- My urologist treated me free of charge for more than a year.

- Vijay guided me into the possibility of hope. He helped me get connected with the companies that provided commission-based work.

- The manager at the employment agency went beyond the limit set by the agency by awarding me a $10,000 grant for my certification.

- Jeff saved my job at his own expense.

- Ben allowed me into his house every day to be trained.

- David and Lisa helped me in so many ways.

Although I was grateful to each and every one at the time, I didn't learn the bigger and higher lessons that our goals and visions should include not just ourselves but other human beings since we are all connected. I was still self- centered and focused on my material goals.

I Left Flagstaff to Reach the Place of My Dreams, Falls Church, VA

I had stayed in Flagstaff for a year and a half. I felt guilty for resigning from my job—Jeff and all the team members had been so helpful to me. In my heart, I felt obligated to them because I wouldn't be a very good technician if it weren't for all those great coworkers. In my heart, I wanted to stay and contribute to Jeff, my team members, and Sears.

But in my mind, I wanted to move to the Virginia and Washington, D.C. area and make $80,000 to $100,000 a year. I was motivated to fulfill my dreams of driving a red Mustang convertible, wearing nice clothes, and eating delicious spicy food. I went through lots of discomfort and tussle between my heart and mind. It wasn't an easy decision for me to make. In the end, my mind won and my heart lost. I left my Sears job after giving a month's notice to Jeff. Jeff, Ben, and David were all sad to see me leave, but they were happy for me. Greg said to me, "Go make your millions."

I was happy that my fears about my old Toyota proved wrong—it turned out to be a reliable car. I arrived in Falls Church, VA in April 2008. The drive was roughly 2,000 miles. Life never ceases to amaze me—I couldn't and didn't expect that old Corolla could last five years, including two long trips from Ypsilanti, MI to Flagstaff, AZ and then finally Flagstaff, AZ to Falls Church, VA. Furthermore, I was able to use the same old car for work, driving it to customers' houses to provide in-home service for an additional year and a half.

My Hopes and Dreams Turned into Misery

Be careful what you wish for.

I was full of hope and excitement on my way to Virginia. However, I found out that there is a huge difference between a dream and reality.

Working as a subcontractor is not the same as working for Sears—I had to gain the trust of customers, I had to explain the problem with the appliance, how I was going to repair it, and how much it was going to cost them. While working at Sears, all I had to do was punch in the job code in my laptop and the price showed up. That was it, since most people trust Sears.

As a subcontractor, I had to sell the repair job, and I could never tell the whole truth to certain cheap customers. I even rode with an experienced subcontractor for a year so that I could learn the art and science of being a subcontractor. He used and abused me—I would carry his tools and perform his job for merely $50 a day, all day until 10 p.m. at night while he made all the money.

Let me elaborate my point by taking you into the reality of one of the days in what I hoped would be my dream world. I wake up in the morning anxious and fearful of living yet another day. I receive a phone call from the owner of the company I worked with before I even had breakfast—and when I say breakfast, I mean having two pieces of toast with black tea. He informs me that I have a total of four jobs for the day, two of which are recalls. I feel awful hearing about recalls because I have to spend more time, more labor, and more driving for jobs I thought were complete.

I go upstairs into the kitchen to prepare black tea only to find that the kitchen is occupied by another tenant. I have to wait 15 minutes while thinking about unpleasant stuff such as recalls and stressful driving. I go into the kitchen to prepare my breakfast. As soon as I have finished, I start heading to my first job, which happens to be a recall in the Haymarket area, which is 35 miles from where I exist miserably.

At the Haymarket residence, I had initially fixed the refrigerator cooling problem by replacing the relay on the compressor. When I arrive at the Haymarket residence for the recall, I find that now the refrigerator has a completely different problem of not producing ice.

The industry standard labor and part warranty covered only the same problem for 90 days, but this was a different problem. The customer happens to be a mean and unreasonable person and has threatened us, saying that if we don't fix the ice production problem he is going to dispute the credit card payment he made the day before. Therefore, I am forced to replace the brand-new ice maker free of charge. I am angry because the job I performed the day before fixed that problem, and it is not fair to force someone to repair something free of charge. Should I go on?

Long story short, I lose money and time on the second recall as well. You almost always lose money and time on recalls because this is the nature of recalls. The best you can do is to minimize the ratio of recalls. Yes, I make some money that day on two fresh jobs, but in the end I break even.

I arrive home after a long and stressful day hoping for peace of mind. But peace of mind is not for me even at home, since the landlady is nosy and bothersome. As soon I enter my room, she complains about my car leaking oil in the driveway. To be fair, she is right. But I am not in a position to buy a new car or even another used car. I simply don't have the money. Therefore, I have an argument with her before I go to bed.

Sorrow Never Comes Alone

I didn't have medical insurance, since I couldn't possibly afford to buy it. Subcontractors aren't usually covered through the companies they work for. Therefore, I was not able to see a psychiatrist or psychotherapist.

Have you noticed that I wasn't taking any dietary and herbal supplements?

As a matter of fact, I didn't take any dietary and herbal supplements for two years from the time I arrived in the Virginia and Washington, D.C. area. I don't know why I didn't do that. I suppose my days were long and nights were short and my mind was occupied with so many problems that I couldn't think right.

Was I Able to Make $80,000 to $100,000 a Year? I Wish

After factoring in my cost of living and my job expenses—tolls, gas, car repairs, etc.—I was bringing in about $22,000 to $25,000 annually, about a quarter of what I'd been expecting to make.

I barely survived renting a room with a shared bathroom and kitchen for two years. It was an awful experience—I sometimes had to wait just for a turn to use the bathroom or kitchen. At least I had lived comfortably and separately in my own apartment in Flagstaff.

Though it is common for adults to have roommates and shared living areas, especially in big, expensive cities, I found that I was negatively impacted by the energy of the people I shared space with. It just wasn't the ideal living situation for me, and that made me feel more miserable. Home should have been a peaceful sanctuary for me, but this particular situation wasn't. Instead, it added to my stress.

At least I learned something about myself and what I could and couldn't tolerate in a living situation.

The traffic patterns were difficult in this metropolitan area as highways got jammed and stayed jammed. I used to get lost because I didn't know the area and GPS navigation used to give slow and vague directions. These driving complications increased my gas and car expenses because I was on the road longer and idling for long periods of time.

It was really hard for me to keep focusing on my dream because I was feeling miserable about my reality.

What are the lessons to be learned?

- Learn to be happy in the now, not in the distant future when you think you will achieve your dream job or buy your house or get married.

- Have goals and vision, but your vision must include others and it should not be a self-centered vision.

Did I learn my lessons? Hell no. It took me many years to learn higher and spiritual lessons nature had been trying to teach me. I was miserable, frustrated and getting angry. I wished many times that I hadn't left Flagstaff for Virginia. Little did I know at the time, things were only going to get worse.

CHAPTER 4

How I Discovered Peace in Nature

How I Discovered Peace in Nature

On July 2011, I went to a customer's house in Fairfax, VA to repair three appliances: a dryer, a refrigerator, and a dishwasher. I diagnosed the problems on all three appliances and provided the customer with the diagnoses. I informed them that I would provide the estimate on all three appliances the next day after finding out about the parts needed to complete the job. I phoned the customer the next day and provided the estimate of $1,149 for all three appliances and he approved the estimate right away.

I ordered the parts needed and picked them up three days later and headed toward the customer's house after informing him that I was on my way. I was driving 40 miles per hour down the customer's street, where the speed limit was 15 miles per hour, and as soon as I arrived at the customer's house, his neighbor came out yelling at me for driving too fast. Naturally, he was concerned and fearful for his kid's safety. We had an argument, which I could have avoided easily by being polite and tactful or by not driving so fast in the neighborhood to begin with.

I was anxious and in a hurried state of mind. I tried to proceed with the repairs on all three appliances, but I was so angry and disturbed that I screwed up. Like most people, there is almost no way I could do anything productive while angry. I was not able to finish my job and it was passed on to another technician. Of course, I lost the money.

I don't know about you, but anger has cost me more than money. I am pretty sure we all have bruised or broken relationships because something we said or did in the heat of the moment.

It wasn't until I discovered something called forest bathing that I finally began to get control of my anger so that I could respond to situations rather than react to them.

Forest Bathing

The idea of forest bathing was started back in 1982 by a Japanese health program to combat work-related stress. The Japanese practice of Shinrin-yoku essentially means forest bathing. In some fields of alternative treatment, forest bathing is considered a form of medicine, as stated by Philip Barr, a Duke University physician who specializes in integrative therapies.[25]

How I Accidentally Discovered Forest Bathing

It was around April 2012 when nature blessed me with a sense of peace by accident. I was in despair, providing in-home appliance repair services in the Virginia and Washington, D.C. area. I was working nine hours a day, six days a week doing a job I was not passionate about at all. I was stressed out, driving around 200 miles a day in chaotic and mostly jammed traffic. I was annoyed, irritable, and angry.

Because I had a negative attitude, I was attracting negative, stingy, and difficult customers. Moreover, I was encountering other problems on a regular basis such as vehicle breakdowns, hitting traffic, and getting parking tickets. Who says the law of attraction doesn't work? It works both ways, and we attract not what we want, wish, or desire but according to our vibrations. By the way, the law of vibration is the primary law, the law of attraction is the secondary law.

As Bob Proctor writes in his book *You Were Born Rich*:

According to the Law of Vibration, everything vibrates or moves; nothing sits idle. Everything is in a constant state of motion, therefore, there is no such thing as "inertia," or a state of rest. "Rate of vibration" is called "frequencies," and the higher the frequency the more potent the force. Thought is the highest form of vibration and since we humans have the ability to think, we can create by means of it.[26]

I used to come home, take a shower, and eat whatever food I could easily get my hands on. After that, I started to watch movies almost every evening until I went to bed, sometimes falling asleep watching movies. Come to think of it, that was all the pleasure I had in my life those days. I had accepted that this was the reality of my life. I became indifferent. I would have arguments with customers almost every day.

One day I came home upset and angry from work as usual. Surprisingly, I decided to go to a neighborhood park—I don't know why I decided to do that. There was a small park located only five minutes walking distance from where I lived. I went there and sat down on the park bench under the trees for around 40 minutes. I didn't do anything else. I had neither an agenda nor any expectation.

I started to feel my body relax in a way I hadn't experienced before. I sort of slipped into a meditative trance induced by natural surroundings. I had a relatively peaceful sleep that night and woke up in an unusually better mood. I had no idea what exactly happened, but I definitely liked the way I felt in the park. I decided to go back to the park the next day and sat down for around 35 minutes. I noticed my body started to feel relaxed and I also felt a pleasant natural sensation that I can't describe in words.

From that day onward I enthusiastically started this practice of going to the park and sitting down quietly for around 40 minutes. I kept practicing consistently for 30 days. The practice of quietly sitting down in the park and paying mindful attention to my surroundings created a shift in my perception. The feeling of anger died down and I wasn't reacting to customers and traffic as much.

My routines and habits changed with regard to my activities when I arrived home from work. I was looking forward to being peaceful. I would come home eagerly, shower quickly and eat my dinner gratefully. After that, I would sit down in the same park for 60 minutes. I started spending more time there just because it made me feel peaceful.

Spending time in nature gives us a sense of clarity, peace, and connections. However, most of us are stuck inside with our focus on electronic devices, such as computers and cell phones. No wonder modern society is faced with all sorts of diseases. Don't get me wrong, I still had stress and frustration from all the driving and an unfulfilling job, but the quality of my life had improved just by allowing me to be in nature.

I was surprised to discover the peacefulness I experienced just by spending some time in nature. I started doing some research online about the healing power of nature on human beings. That is how I found out about the practice of forest bathing. I had already been practicing it, I just didn't know what I had been doing is called forest bathing, and I didn't know the research behind it.

What is Forest Bathing Anyway?

Forest bathing is about connecting to yourself through nature. It is immersing yourself in the myriad of sensory pleasures of the forest. It is an act of allowing scents, sights, and sounds to let us immerse in natural surroundings.

Hiking, rock climbing, and even walking in nature is not forest bathing, because forest bathing is an act of being, not doing.

You don't even need a forest to practice forest bathing—all you need is to find a spot in a local park without lots of noise and activity.

Research has shown that the practice of forest bathing offers many physiological as well as psychological benefits. Here is a list of clinically-documented results: [27]

1. Alleviating depression

2. Better sleep

3. Increased mental clarity

4. Boosted mood

5. Increased immune function_

6. Normalization of blood pressure

7. Chronic pain relief

8. Lowering levels of cortisol

All these awesome benefits made me ask this important question: Is there a physically identifiable process or action in the forest that carries the healing power? The answer is yes. Many plants and trees produce phytoncides (wood essential oils) to protect them from afflictions.

Scientific studies have shown that phytoncide can be beneficial to human beings as well. Cedar, garlic, locust, oak, onion, pine, tea tree, and many other plants give off phytoncides. They are emitted from the trees and plants into the forest atmosphere. When humans breathe in these compounds, they gain the wonderful healing and protective benefits of phytoncides.[28]

How Nature Helped Me Feel Grateful

Most of us know that it feels peaceful to be grateful. Some of us write in a gratitude journal either early in the morning or just before bedtime. But the challenge is how to actually *feel* grateful—at least it was a challenge for me. Again, nature came to my aid.

This is how I developed the habit of being grateful and actually generating feelings of gratitude. I started walking 30 minutes a day, five days a week. I used to go to a local lake with lots of trees in the fall season. I started appreciating the beauty of the lake and trees while smelling the aroma of different plants and trees while I was strolling. I used to go into a meditative trance with sights, sounds, and smells of the whole scene and I felt grateful.

The idea was to cultivate gratitude regularly so that gratitude becomes my habit, and it did. I became a more grateful person. Being human, I still get jealous, bitter, resentful, and angry, but the intensity and frequency have decreased and I feel like I can handle those emotions better so they don't take over my day or life.

Forest Bathing Tips I Learned from My Experience

- You really don't need to go too far. I found a place to practice forest bathing that was only a five minute walk from where I lived. Some of you may need to go farther than that depending on how far you live from a local park.

- You don't need to spend 60 minutes or even 40 minutes practicing forest bathing—you can go for only 20 minutes and still derive mental and physical benefits. But it feels good, so you might, like I did, start spending even more time in nature.

- Forest bathing means listening, not talking. I always practiced forest bathing alone. But if you go with others, agree to spend time in silence. You can't talk and perceive the sensory pleasures of nature at the same time.

- Don't have an agenda. This can be harder for some individuals, but remember that forest bathing is about being, not doing.

- You should try to awaken your sense of touch when you're forest bathing. You can do this in many ways. My favorite way is walking barefoot on the grass.

- Turn off your cellphone.

Forest Bathing in the Fall and Spring

I find it very pleasurable to practice forest bathing in the fall and spring seasons because the sights, sounds, and smells, especially the smells of these seasons, make me go into a meditative trance. These are my favorite seasons.

I have the luxury to practice forest bathing in the morning, in the evening, or the afternoon, depending on my schedule. The benefit of forest bathing in the evening is that I become relaxed and peaceful and usually get a restful night's sleep. On the other hand, it helps my day go more smoothly and I'm more productive if I practice forest bathing in the morning.

Forest Bathing in Winter

You can still practice forest bathing in winter and derive some benefits, despite the fact that most trees and plants don't have leaves, depending on where you live. It depends on how comfortable you are in cold weather and how cold the day actually is when you want to go forest bathing. Moreover, it also depends on where you live, since Minnesota winters are much colder than northern Virginia winters.

The Challenges of Forest Bathing in the Summer

Forest bathing in the summer has some challenges for me, since I've never liked heat, humidity, or scorching sun. Comparatively speaking, I don't feel as good in summer. It's not just heat and humidity that annoys me, but also bugs and insects. I only use plant-based lemon eucalyptus bug spray, but it's only partially effective.

I still practice forest bathing in summer despite all these challenges, but not as much compared to fall, spring, and winter. Incidentally, I have had the most arguments with customers and other people in the summer, since I don't feel good and tend to react to people, events, and circumstances easily.

Since I was not able to completely control my mood or **my anger** with the help of forest bathing in the summer, I decided to try anger management in April 2020.

Anger Management

I participated in seven individual sessions with a therapist who specializes in anger management. The goal was to manage my anger. I learned some skills. The first thing was to know exactly what anger is.

What Is Anger, Anyway?

Anger is the feeling or emotion that ranges from mild irritation to intense fury and rage.[29] There is a difference between anger and aggression. Aggression is a behavior that is intended to cause harm or injury to another person or damage to property.[30] Anger, on the other hand, is about a set of attitudes that motivates aggressive behavior. Anger can be viewed as a maladaptive habit when anger is displayed frequently and aggressively.

A maladaptive habit is described as a pattern of inflexible behavior that reflects poorly on self-control. These behaviors occur despite the known harmful consequences. The term describes behaviors that modify, adapt, or adjust poorly.[31] Having angry outbursts, flying into a rage, and becoming so angry that it can lead to aggression are considered maladaptive behaviors because of the lack of self-control. Most people know these behaviors are problematic, but they still cause harm with their anger.

Anger Monitoring

According to the Substance Abuse and Mental Health Services Administration (SAMHSA), there are two ways to monitor anger.[32] The first way to monitor anger is by using a 1 to 10 scale called the anger meter. A score of 1 on the anger meter represents lack of anger whereas 10 represent explosive loss of control over anger.

A second important way to monitor anger is to identify the signs that occur while anger is increasing. These signs serve as a warning that anger is escalating. There are four categories:

1. Physical

2. Emotional

3. Behavioral

4. Cognitive[33]

I Gained Awareness about My Anger

As human beings, we all get angry from time to time. But anger became a problem for me for three reasons. First, I got angry too frequently. Second, I was getting angry too intensely. Third, I was expressing anger inappropriately.

For many years, there was a popular belief that aggressive expression of anger, such as beating on pillows, was therapeutic. Recent studies have found that venting anger in an aggressive manner reinforces aggressive behaviors.[34]

According to SAMHSA, an anger episode consists of three phases:

1. Buildup

2. Explosion

3. Aftermath[35]

One of the primary objectives of anger management is to stop you from reaching the explosion phase. I remember I used to lose control when reacting to people—I would automatically explode. I would feel two different ways in the aftermath phase. Sometimes I would feel guilt and shame, while other times I would feel calm after releasing my tension. But I almost always paid the price when I exploded—customers would cancel jobs without even paying what they owed me.

I remember my father used to get really angry, but he became calm afterward. That is how my father released tension—explosive anger helped him do that. We all have patterns that we learned from our parents, whether we like them or not.

Lesson Learned

I learned how to express assertively instead of aggressively. The first step was awareness. I gained awareness about how I usually expressed myself. I also learned about four basic styles of communication:

1. Passive communication

2. Aggressive communication

3. Passive-aggressive communication

4. Assertive communication[36]

Here is a scenario to explain the four types of communication. I provide a customer an estimate of $349 and diagnosis that the main control board is the problem with their dryer. The stingy customer asks me irritating questions such as "Why is the estimate so expensive?" and "Why do you think the main control board is the problem and not the sensor?"

Passive response: I leave the customer's house quietly, as I was instructed to do so by the company owner when faced with irritating questions from stingy customers. The appliance repair company owner knows that I can't handle these types of customers or questions. If I stay and communicate with the customer then there will be a problem and an unhappy customer at the end.

Aggressive response: I am loud and irritated and say "That is what we charge and you can decline the estimate if you think it is expensive. If we are wrong about the control board, then we will pay the price, not you."

Passive-aggressive response: I leave the customer's house quietly but with a body gesture advertising that I am angry.

Assertive response: "Sir, this is the amount we charge for this particular repair. We offer quality service in every way and our rates are competitive in the area. If I am wrong about the control board being the issue, then you don't have to pay for the part or the repair. You are covered for 90 days labor and the part warranty."

I used to either communicate aggressively or passive-aggressively. The goal for any individual is to communicate assertively. It doesn't mean that I always communicate assertively. It simply means I communicate assertively most of the time.

The aspect of anger that anger management lacks is it doesn't go into the root causes of anger. For instance, I didn't learn why I used to get angry so frequently and so intensely in the anger management sessions. Fortunately, I had already discovered my "why," or the source of my anger, back in August of 2019. I took the anger management course in April of 2020 when I already had the awareness I needed about my "why." This allowed me to benefit more from the anger management lessons.

CHAPTER 5

The Best Thing That Ever
Happened to Me

The Best Thing That Ever Happened to Me

I got married on December 10, 2013. I got divorced on May 18, 2018. This was the first and only time I've been married (so far). Right after getting married, I was faced with a crisis. Crises tend to show people who they actually are—their way of being, their way of thinking—if they are willing to invest the time and effort to look within. The crisis made me worried and fearful.

I was worried about how the hell I was going to support my wife on my income when we got married. I was just getting by. I was full of fears, imagining all kinds of scenarios such as getting evicted from my apartment and living on the street, eating from a dumpster. No matter what I did or where I went, my mind was occupied with worry and fear. Come to think of it, I was truly focused for the first time in my life, though my focus was all on negative scenarios.

This crisis came out to be a blessing in disguise because it led to my personal growth journey, which continues to this day. I wouldn't be where I am right now if I didn't get married. Though we lived together miserably as a couple for only 10 months, my marriage was the best thing that ever happened to me.

For that, I am truly grateful for my marriage and to my ex-wife.

You might be asking the obvious questions:

- Why didn't I think about how I was going to support my wife before getting married?

- Why did I decide to get married at 44?

- Why couldn't my wife contribute financially?

I believe the first question is the most important. I was able to answer it eventually, though it took me many years. You see "thinking" is the highest form of function humans can perform. Matter of fact, thinking is what differentiates us from many of the creatures on the planet. Mental activity doesn't constitute thinking.

Bob Proctor quotes Kenneth McFarland as saying the following: "Two percent of people think, three percent of people think they think, and ninety-five percent of people would rather die than think."[37]

I wasn't thinking and I was part of the 95 percent of people. That is the answer to the first question. I was operating on autopilot based on a program that had been installed in my subconscious mind.

To answer the second and third questions we need to dig a little deeper into paradigms.

My Paradigm

According to Bob Proctor, a paradigm is "a mental program that has almost exclusive control over our habitual behaviors," and almost all of our behaviors are habitual.[38]

I was programmed exactly in the same way we all are programmed: both genetically and environmentally. I was the eldest child. My parents would have arguments with each other on a continuous basis about many things including money. I learned as a baby that money was a source of arguments instead of a source of joy.

No wonder I have struggled all my life with money—not just making money but also keeping money. I didn't have much income to begin with, and I then I would lose money because I would have trouble with customers, my car would break down more than usual, and a host of other problems.

Why wasn't I making $80,000 to $100,000 a year being a very good and hard-working technician contractor?

I discovered that no matter how hard and long you work—no matter how smart you are, no matter how much education you have—if you don't have the right mindset, you will not reach your full potential and make the money you want to make.

You might be wondering why I didn't go back to work for a company like Sears after failing to achieve my goal of desired income. Well, although I was really and truly miserable being an appliance repair contractor, I had lots of freedom and flexibility to start my workday when I wanted. The same goes for how and when to end my day. Moreover, I didn't have to wear a uniform. I didn't have to worry that somebody would call the phone number on my truck and complain about my driving just because they had a bad day.

The work environment, work conditions, and the flexibility

were ideal. If only I could find a way to enjoy the work and make more money.

When it comes to customers, the most important thing is how you deal with them, and that means your way of being and doing. I was anxious, confused, and unhappy when providing service to customers. I used to be in a hurry instead of being relaxed and calm. No wonder I was broke, working hard and long, while other technicians were making the kind of money I wanted to be making. Let me illustrate my point with the following incident.

My Way of Reacting to Stingy Customers

In June 2011, I went to a service call to fix a washing machine in a second-floor condo in the city of Burke, Virginia. I diagnosed the problem in the washer to be a leaky water solenoid valve and provided the customers with an estimate of $199 with parts and labor.

I also noticed a very old and brittle hot water hose coming from the plumbing shut-off valve to the washer. I intended to inform the customer once the estimate for the washer job was approved because this brittle hose, though connected to the washer, was not actually a part of the washer. A washer's cold and hot water hoses can be replaced by an appliance repair technician, a plumber, or even a handyman. This was not exactly an appliance repair job.

The customer was cheap and didn't approve the estimate. I was supposed to have customers sign the company invoice before I even touched an appliance to diagnose the problem because it would give both me and the repair company I worked with a waiver from fake and nonsense litigations. Since I was in a hurry and anxious that day I didn't follow procedure and have the customer sign the invoice. The customer even refused to pay the $45 toward service charges, which I earned by getting to the customer's house and providing a written diagnosis.

I had an argument with the customer for about 25 minutes and left his condo without getting the $45 and, of course, without informing the customer about his brittle washer hose.

The very old and brittle water hose burst the following night and flooded not only the customer's condo but the downstairs condo as well. There was a lot of damage to both condos and the customer blamed me and the company I worked with, since I was the last person to touch the appliance.

The water hose was going to burst anytime regardless of me being there, but the customer didn't want to understand or accept the true cause of the accident. My mistake was not getting the customer's signature on the company's invoice, which would waive us and save us from this blame and waste of time.

The customer threatened to sue us, and his downstairs neighbor was taking him to court. Thankfully, I had liability insurance and we let my liability insurance deal with the customer. The bad news was that the insurance company declined to renew my liability insurance the next year. I ended up paying three times more money to get liability insurance from a different company.

I was angry at the customer. I was obsessed with him for being stingy. I realized that my anger was associated with my father, who was also cheap in some ways. Because I rebelled against my father's pattern and way of being, cheap customers used to trigger my anger.

Lessons Learned

- Cheap individuals are out of harmony with the universe and they get to spend more money on losses than they actually save. They also waste their time by causing additional problems.

- I used to get triggered by cheap customers. Now I simply avoid them.

My Idea of Marriage

My subconscious mind equated marriage with suffering and misery, since I almost always saw my parents unhappy. My parents' behavior affected me in two important ways. First, I developed an unhappy personality. Second, I never wanted to get married as I "learned" marriage was a source of suffering.

My parents and siblings asked me for a long time when I was going to get married.

I always said "Never," and I meant it. Therefore, I didn't get married until I was 44.

Let's recap the points I made before answering them:

- I was not able to think right.

- I was unhappy.

- I worked hard and long with ambitions for many years, but failed miserably every single time.

The state of mind, or mindset, is the most important, intangible asset any individual possess. The mindset determines almost everything that goes on in the life of an individual.

States of Mind

1. STATE OF MIND "A"

I used to be excited, ambitious, and focused while I was working toward a goal such as working toward getting a Windows networking job or working toward being an appliance repair contractor.

2. STATE OF MIND "B"

I used to be depressed, angry, bitter, jealous, resentful, and fearful after I failed to achieve a goal. I was literally non-productive and living life with psychiatric medicine.

3. NEWLY ACQUIRED STATE OF MIND "C"

Since 2011, I acquired a new state of mind. This time I was not depressed like I had been in the past. I gave up on anything and everything. I resigned to my fate. I didn't get disappointed because I didn't expect any good thing in my life. What will be will be became my philosophy.

However, I didn't accept my fate of failure and poverty, which I saw as an injustice. I had anger inside of me. The "C" mindset is the combination of accepting (only consciously) my fate and being angry at the same time. It is sort of like you let something into your life without giving it any thought and then you get angry afterward when you see the results.

Your state of mind determines how much success you will achieve, whether it is financial success or success in marriage. The mindset also determines the kind of decisions you make. I was not capable of making the right decisions, and my parents offered their help (just like they had done various times in the past) by offering to find me a bride. I accepted their help, and that is how Saima ended up in my life.

Me and My Wife

I don't intend to badmouth my ex-wife in any way shape or form. The purpose of writing this section is the same as the purpose of writing this book: to share my experiences and the lessons I learned from these experiences in hopes that you might find them beneficial.

Keep in mind, though, that I didn't learn the lessons right away. It took me many years to understand after I gained some level of awareness. Remember that it is not important what happened but what meaning we give to whatever it is that happened—it depends on our perception, which we can develop as we gain a higher level of awareness.

I am going to show you what kind of person she was, and by showing her characteristics I will automatically reveal who I really was at that time in my life. She was angry, unhappy, and greedy.

Is it an accident that we were attracted to each other? There are no accidents in life. Everything happens according to universal laws that govern our lives. My wife and I were vibrating in harmony (in resonance) with each other.

We got married on December 10, 2013, after which it took her more than two years to arrive in the U.S. due to problems with her immigration application. She finally arrived here on February 11, 2016. We only lived together for 10 months before getting separated on January 9, 2017. Looking back, I am fully convinced that our marriage was destined to fall apart.

It is not what I did and didn't do and how she reacted—the real reason was much deeper. The foundation of our marriage was faulty, lacking trust and sincerity. I was just as responsible for that as she was. She married me because she thought I would be making lots of money being an appliance repair contractor. As for me, I married her without giving it any thought to what it meant to be married.

Since I'd never wanted to get married, I hadn't considered the responsibilities of marriage. Other than thinking that marriage brings misery, which is why I didn't want to get married in the first place, I didn't know anything about marriage.

At first, my wife didn't get a job because she didn't speak English. I had her enrolled in an English class, and I wanted her to focus on finishing the class so she could apply for better jobs rather than working the low-income jobs she qualified for.

I was finally able to help her get a job at Safeway after about nine months. She kept her income to herself and didn't want me knowing how much she was making.

There were incidents that happened between us that didn't help the situation. She blamed me for her visa problems. Then our child died prematurely before birth. She blamed me because I was not with her when it happened. I felt awful and stayed home for a couple days.

As far as I remember, I never had confidence when I was in the relationship. I had been living with fears and worries since the day I got married. If anything, my fears and worries had been multiplied after observing her patterns and behaviors of anger, unhappiness, and complaining. I had been thinking and considering my options of increasing my income.

I had seen individuals working longer hours to increase their income. I could have easily gotten more service calls if I wanted to go that route. But it wasn't possible for me to work longer hours physically or mentally. I used to get triggered easily by negative customers, customers who asked a lot of nonsense questions, and customers who were stingy.

Lacking in customer skills wasn't my only challenge, though it was the one major challenge. I would get stressed out and angry in traffic jams. I would screw up easily if I went to a customer's house right after coming out of a traffic jam. There is no way I could work longer hours fixing appliances. I was thinking about doing a second job, but it was not feasible. First, I didn't have any education or any skills. Second, I was physically and mentally exhausted. I didn't have any energy.

Therefore, the best option was for me to grow myself mentally though a personal growth program.

How My Marriage Led to My Personal Growth

I went through a lot of misery and suffering during my marriage until we finally got divorced in 2018. I believe I had to go through suffering and misery to learn the lessons I needed to learn. I didn't suffer in vain. My marriage helped me in so many ways:

- Being married made me realize what exactly I wanted and didn't want in my future marriage.

- I realized that it is not enough to have the desire for a happy spouse—I needed to be happy to attract a happy partner.

- I started a personnel growth journey while I was married, although I didn't have any intention to grow as person. My only goal was to make more money so that I could support our family.

- I started to gain awareness slowly but surely while still married. Nature guided me through hunches and impulses which I received while I was married.

Here is how the process of transformation started:

I really liked the movie *The Secret,* so much so that I watched it 11 times. My therapist in Flagstaff recommended it to me, but I didn't watch it until 2012. I got excited and hopeful every time I watched it, but I never figured out how to apply the principles into my life.

One day I was inspired to watch it again after waking up in the night. I really didn't want to watch it again because I already watched it so many times, but for some reason I followed my hunch.

As soon as I started watching it I had a second hunch: I needed to write down the names of teachers who appeared in the movie. I wrote down the names Bob Proctor, Jack Canfield, John Assarraf, among others. Once I got all these names, I started researching them online. Keep in mind that I didn't plan anything—I was sort of automatically taking one step after another.

I Started My Personal Growth Journey with Bob Proctor

Once I learned about Bob Proctor's company, the Proctor Gallagher Institute (PGI), I enrolled in an inexpensive program called "Six Minutes to Success."[39] The way it worked was I would get a six minute video delivered to my email every morning. I continued with the program for around three months.

I had an impulse to grow in a bigger way instead of just watching a six-minute video every day. I called and set up an over-the-phone consultation with PGI's sales manager. After discussing PGI's programs and my needs, I decided to go with Bob Proctor's 12-month coaching program.[40]

Facing Multiple Challenges

Although I decided to go with the 12-month coaching program

with Bob Proctor, I didn't have any money, let alone $7,000, which is the total cost of the program.

Let me elaborate my financial situation. Not only had I spent a reasonable sum toward getting married (airfare, clothing, marriage ceremonies, etc.) but I also took two months off from work to get ready for marriage and the ceremonies. This was the first challenge I faced toward starting my growth journey. PGI offered me a four-payment installment plan and I made the first payment with a credit card.

The second challenge was even bigger than the first. Although I decided in my conscious mind to go with the coaching program, I was not comfortable with the idea of investing such a large sum on a personal development program. I couldn't sleep a few nights thinking about it. I contacted the sales manager and informed him that I wanted to quit. He said, "Let me get Bob Proctor to explain to you the benefits of this coaching program, and if you are still not convinced then I will have your payment refunded."

I was excited to hear Bob Proctor over the phone the next day. He said, "Take my words and this program will change your life if you let it."

I changed my mind and decided to stay with the coaching program.

Bob Proctor's 12-Month Coaching Program

The 12-month program is PGI's most extensive program. It is divided into 12 modules and covers so many topics and lessons. I would participate in live webinars and Q&A sessions held by Bob Proctor himself.

I gained knowledge about many things, though I didn't fully understand them yet. Knowledge refers to *information gained* through education. On the other hand, once understanding is acquired through experience, then it can be applied to improve lives.

The essence of the knowledge I gained can be summed up in these three points:

1. How I had been conditioned or programmed both genetically and environmentally.

2. Why I was getting the results I was getting (financial, physical, mental, etc.).

3. How I could change my way of thinking or conditioning, and subsequently change the results I was getting.

I did all that I could do to follow Bob Proctor's directions. I listened to recordings of the webinars over and over again. I read the books he recommended.

As far as results were concerned, I was not able to improve my life. In a sense I was still sick, unhappy, and making the same amount of money I used to make before I started the coaching program. It is because I had suffered many physical and emotional traumas in my life, and emotional healing was needed so that mental blocks could be removed.

However, the most important thing I gained is an understanding that I can actually improve my life and live a happy, healthy, and wealthy life. I realized that I have the power within. My personal growth journey had started.

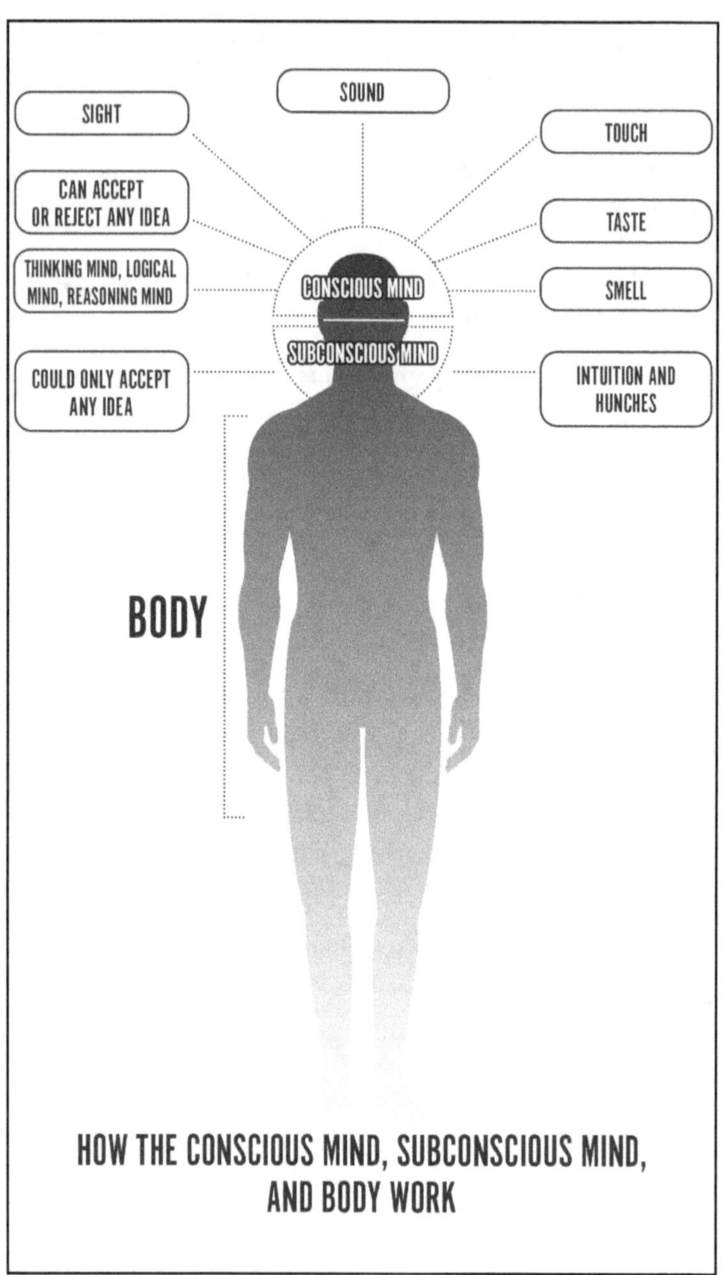

HOW THE CONSCIOUS MIND, SUBCONSCIOUS MIND,
AND BODY WORK

We have only one mind, but our mind possesses two distinctive characteristics. The dividing line between the two is well known to all thinking individuals. The conscious mind is a thinking mind or logical mind or reasoning mind and functions with the five physical senses. The conscious mind gives us an ability to either accept or reject any idea or thought.

By using the conscious mind correctly, we can think correctly and deposit the truth in the subconscious mind (the subconscious mind can only accept an idea). The great aspiration, inspirations, and vision for a grander life comes from the subconscious mind. Our subconscious speaks to us in intuitions, impulses, hunches, and ideas, and it is always telling us to grow and transcend to greater and greater heights because the subconscious is in touch with infinite intelligence. The body is the instrument of mind. [41]

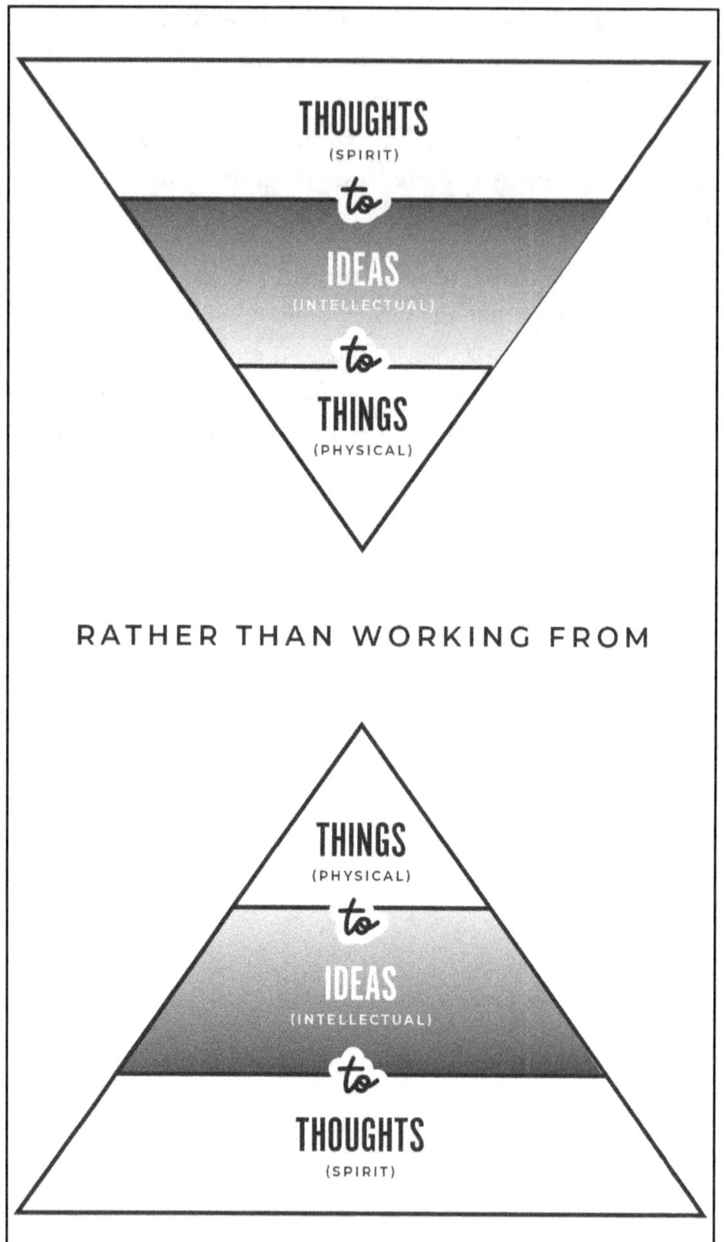
THOUGHTS
(SPIRIT)
to
IDEAS
(INTELLECTUAL)
to
THINGS
(PHYSICAL)
RATHER THAN WORKING FROM
THINGS
(PHYSICAL)
to
IDEAS
(INTELLECTUAL)
to
THOUGHTS
(SPIRIT)

We are spiritual beings living in physical bodies. We have to use our intuition while building an idea instead of the five physical senses. When we rely too much on our physical senses, then we ignore intuition or gut feelings. How many times have you ignored a gut feeling and later thought, "I should have paid attention to my feelings"?

CHAPTER 6

Food Healed My Body and Mind

Food Healed My Body and Mind

After separating from my wife in January 2017, I sometimes got overwhelmed with the feelings of confusion, regret, guilt, and even anger. Although I never questioned my decision to get separated, as I believed that was the right decision for both of us, the way we did it caused suffering for both of us.

All the suffering and pain taught me many lessons, which I believe I had to go through to become who I am today. My victim mindset kept asking me the same question: "Why do I have to go though some sort of suffering?"

Although I had already started my personal growth journey in June 2015, I still didn't know how to deal with all this. One evening I was searching for a favorite movie to watch—my favorites are old movies from the `50s and `60s, and they usually lift me out of negative feelings. While I was searching, my eyes caught a documentary called Hungry for Change.[42]

I wasn't used to watching documentaries of any kind because they didn't make me feel joyful and happy. But for some unknown reason I skeptically selected *Hungry for Change* and started watching. I really liked it and it changed my perception of food and made me realize how important a healthy diet is.

I became obsessed with other documentaries on food such as *Forks over Knives*.[43] I started doing research on how food could make me healthier and happier.

What Is Epigenetic?

The Centers for Disease Control and Prevention defines epigenetic the following way:

> Our genes play an important role in our health, but so do our behaviors and environment, such as what we eat and how physically active, we are. Epigenetic is the study of how our behaviors and environment can cause changes that affect the way our genes work. Unlike genetics, epigenetic changes are reversible and do not change our DNA sequence, but they can change how our body reads a DNA sequence. Genetic changes affect gene expression to turn "ON" and "OFF" and our diet can cause epigenetic changes, making a clear connection between what we eat and our health.[44]

Food Is the Most Powerful Medicine

The line between medicine and food is thinner than most of us realize. Both go into our bodies, where they affect our overall health. Food has turned out to be a more powerful medicine than we were taught.

Food contains information that speaks to our environment and genes, programming our bodies with messages of health and happiness or sickness and misery. Although what we eat doesn't change the sequence of our DNA, our diet has a profound effect on how our genes express the possibilities encoded in our DNA.[45] Good health starts at the end of our fork. We need to realize and utilize the power of food to help our society overcome epidemics of chronic diseases.

The way we produce and consume food is at the center of most of our health, environmental and economic crises. Although I care about our environment, I will stay focused on human health.

There are diet wars going on, such as low-fat vegan versus high-fat paleo. The disagreement mostly centers around the moral issue of eating meat, not on human health concerns. I respect what vegetarians believe and hope they respect what I believe.

Nowadays more and more people know that a good diet is the cornerstone of health, but are confused about what to eat and what to not eat. I follow the practices of Dr. Mark Hyman.

Dr. Mark Hyman is leading a health revolution. He is a practicing family physician recognized internationally for being a leader, speaker, educator, and advocate in the field of functional medicine. Dr. Hyman is the founder and director of The UltraWellness Center, the Head of Strategy and Innovation of the Cleveland Clinic Center for Functional Medicine, a fourteen-time *New York Times* bestselling author, and Board President for Clinical Affairs for The Institute for Functional Medicine. He also hosts the podcast *The Doctor's Farmacy*.[46]

Dr. Hyman is one the most important voices in the world of medicine, health, and nutrition. He has helped thousands of people lead happier and healthier lives. He lays out dietary plans that are delicious, nutritious, sustainable, and satisfying to taste buds. He provides an elegant insight into the confusing world of fat by explaining that the right fat can be a powerful addition to any diet. He offers not just an opinion, but clear-headed descriptions, expert analysis, and effective solutions for anybody to follow and improve their health. Inspired by his work, I came up with the mantra, "I am always aware of my intention with the food I am about to eat or drink."

I always ask this insightful question before I consume any food: "Why the hell am I consuming this?" In my opinion, we eat food for three different reasons:

1. We eat food because we are simply hungry.

2. We eat food to nourish our body. (Unfortunately, most of us don't eat for that reason.)

3. We eat to seek pleasure. (YouTube is full of videos from all over the world showing us countless dishes and countless ways to enjoy our food. The whole restaurant industry has thrived because they offer delicious food, whether or not it is nutritional. I eat for pleasure only occasionally.)

My Dietary Practices

I added healthy foods such as seeds, nuts, vegetables, and fruits to my diet. However, I didn't completely transform my diet. Here is a list of my general rules for eating:

- I skip a meal if I am angry or upset, because my body will not be able to digest food properly. I just drink a fruit smoothie or eat nuts and seeds on those occasions.

- I don't watch TV or movies while I eat. I eat quietly and gratefully.

- I eat sprouted bread at breakfast instead of flour bread. Sprouted bread is made from whole grains that have begun to sprout or germinate. With proper moisture and warmth, whole grain seeds begin to sprout into a plant. According to Melissa Groves, "The sprouting process offers several nutrition benefits, compared to breads made from unsprouted grains or grain flours."[47]

- I drink plenty of water, roughly seventy to one hundred ounces (12.5 cups) a day.

- I usually don't drink soda, and if I get to drink it, I drink regular soda and not diet soda, because diet contains artificial sweeteners, which are addictive.

- I limit my caffeine intake by drinking my favorite black tea only at breakfast.

- I avoid eating deep fried food, especially at dinner, because it is hard to digest while I sleep.

- I drink freshly made vegetable juice instead of fruit juice. Commercially sold fruit juice, whether apple, orange, or grape or even a fancy blend, is high in sugar. An eight-ounce serving of juice and cola contains about 30 grams of sugar on average and that comes to about eight teaspoons.[48]

After changing my diet I saw noticeable results in as little as three weeks. I started experiencing feelings of pleasure, alertness, and calmness. We humans can have many feelings at the same time, and as such I still had feelings of regret, confusion, and guilt arising from my separation, but I was able to deal with those feelings easier.

Lessons Learned

I started to behave better once I was feeling better, despite the cognitive distortion that existed in my mind. What does that mean?

It means a healthy diet helped me experience positive emotions as long as nothing triggered me.

A trigger is an outside stimulus that can be a person, condition, or circumstance. A trigger is usually negative stimulus because we usually react instead of respond to people, conditions, and circumstances.

I used to react to stingy customers far too easily prior to eating a healthy diet. For instance, I went to a stingy customer's house to repair his refrigerator. I provided an estimate after diagnosing the problem. He asked question after question and then didn't approve the estimate. I was triggered and reacted by yelling at him. He threw me out of his house and complained to my manager.

These behaviors were counterproductive. However, after feeling better with the help of my healthy diet, I started to behave better. It wasn't a perfect solution, but it was a step.

It had been around four months since I improved my dietary habits and I had been feeling and behaving better when my younger brother came from London, England and moved in with me. This was in April of 2017.

He was an angry and negative person, much like I used to be. I let him move in because he was my brother. We started having arguments the day he arrived. We had been arguing at least three times a week. There were certain issues that caused the arguments on a consistent basis, such as me watching TV too loudly and the apartment being too cold for him. There were new issues that kept arising regularly between us.

I was between a rock and hard place. I couldn't ask him to move out because I knew if I did he would never forgive me, regardless of who was right. I tried, but I wasn't able to make temporary living arrangements that we both could live with. Moreover, our parents and siblings were getting informed about our situation, so it was not easy to hide.

For instance, my mother would call, and if I sounded upset then she would sense that something was not right with me. She would know what was going on after asking questions. They were concerned that the situation could get out of control in the heat of the moment.

He moved out after living with me for five months. I was physically and mentally exhausted, and so was he. My job also suffered during this time. I earned almost 40 percent less than I was earning before. My recall rate on the job I completed almost doubled.

Bigger Lessons Learned

A healthy diet plays a major role in the health and happiness of an individual.

But a healthy diet is not enough to maintain health and happiness, especially when we are faced with bigger challenges. Challenges are part of life and we cannot avoid them. We need healthy paradigms and the right mindset. Yes, my brother had a bad temper and negative attitude, but I didn't have to react to him and his behaviors the way I did.

I realized in early 2021 that we needed to work on all the following areas to live a happy and healthy life:

1. Thoughts that empower us. ("A man's life is what his thoughts make of it.")[49]

2. A healthy diet

3. Our connections to nature

4. Getting six to eight hours of peaceful sleep

5. Social connections, including love

6. Living life with purpose

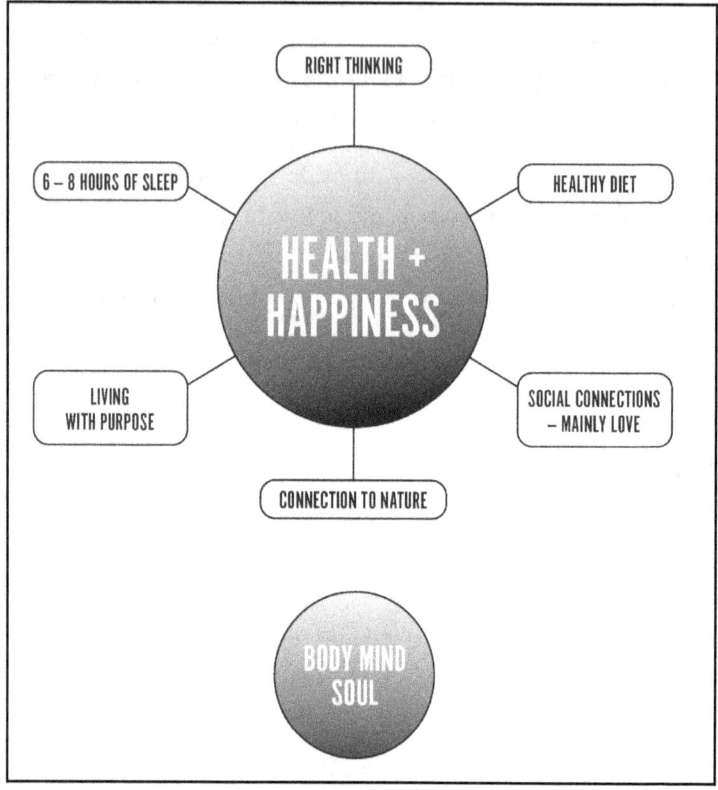

CHAPTER 7

How I Turned My Challenges
into Opportunities

How I Turned My Challenges into Opportunities

Accumulation of Personal Debt

We are faced with challenges throughout our lives. The way we face those challenges dictate our outcomes, and our paradigms dictate our ways of facing those challenges.

The biggest challenge I was faced with was the accumulation of my personal debt. By 2020 I had managed to accumulate the highest level of debt I'd ever had in my life. I had some credit card debt that had started piling up since 2016. Then I almost doubled my debt in 2017. My debt continued to increase in 2018 and 2019 until eventually reaching its highest level near the end of 2019.

However, I never felt guilty about my debt at all. It was a catch-22. For me to live a happy, healthy, and prosperous life I had to improve my beliefs and paradigms. In order to improve my beliefs and paradigms, I had to invest money. Since I didn't have any money, I had to borrow money using credit cards. The other choice I had was to keep living a miserable existence. Therefore, I made the conscious decision to go that route, but I still had been getting stressed out about my personal debt.

That's not to say I was comfortable with this huge amount of debt. We all have different comfort zones with regard to personal debt, and this amount of debt went far beyond my comfort zone. Moreover, I had fears about credit card debt from my past experiences. I was forced to file for bankruptcy in 2002 because I wasn't able to manage my debt properly. I still remember the unpleasant memories I experienced in the aftermath of the bankruptcy process— anything requiring a credit check presented challenges, like leasing an apartment or getting a cell phone contract. I think people who go through the bankruptcy experience and its aftermath can understand my point much easier. I learned my lesson about credit card debt the hard way and any lesson you learn the hard way you will not forget.

I Was Betting on Myself, Not on Lottery Tickets and Casinos

I gained an understanding through reading inspirational books and personal growth material that I could actually improve my health, happiness, and income by improving my beliefs and paradigms. I had no idea exactly how long it was going to take for me to see and enjoy my results. I thought it would happen sooner, but I was dead wrong. It took much longer than I could imagine. But the important thing is improvement in my life did occur for me and everybody else to see.

Not only was I happy investing my money, time, and effort in personal development, I was also obsessed with it.

Investing Money and Time on My Personal Growth

From January 2016 to June 2017, I invested considerable sums of money to building my online business on Amazon's platform. Unfortunately, I had to use my credit cards because I didn't have any money. I failed miserably in the end, but I learned a lot from my mistakes. My business endeavor failed, but I grew as an individual.

In August 2019, I participated in the Hoffman Process[50] on borrowed money using an installment program, using my credit card to pay for those installments. The Hoffman organization provided me a grant, for which I am grateful, but I still had to invest a decent sum toward their fees plus toward transport and lodging (participants are encouraged to stay two days alone before returning to their usual residence or family).

I learned an important lesson of maintaining good credit from my unpleasant past experience. I was reaping the benefits of my good credit history.

The Great Intangible Asset (Good Credit History)

Although good credit history is an intangible asset, it is a great asset to have. I managed my credit card debt well, thanks to my good credit history, which I had rebuilt after my financial difficulties in 2001. I kept my credit debt at 0 percent APR by transferring my credit card balances from one credit card to another on a yearly basis, since 0 percent APR period usually ends in one year. All I had to pay were 3 percent balance transfer fees on my total credit card balance every year. The major reason I was able to build my good credit history is I learned my lessons from having awful credit history.

The more awareness you acquire, the more ways you'll be shown how to improve your life. That's how you keep moving forward.

Yearly Performance Evaluation

Starting in December 2017, I began evaluating my performance on a yearly basis at the end of each year. I looked at both my tangible and intangible accomplishments. I also pondered the mistakes I made and failures I suffered and more importantly the lessons I learned from all these mistakes and failures.

When I was doing my yearly performance evaluation in December 2019, I noticed that I grew to be a happier and healthier person. But I also realized that my credit card debt had been growing since January 2016 and it was now the highest it had ever been. I was fearful and worried that this personal debt could and would become unmanageable if it kept growing at this rate. I realized I had to do something, but I had no idea what I could possibly do.

I had been trying to increase my income since June 2015 without any success. I started on my personal development journey for the sole reason of increasing my income. Unfortunately, I was focused on my personal debt and vibrating on debt vibration. Not good at all.

Debt Mental Block

While I had been successfully managing my credit card debt at 0 percent APR, I developed a debt mental block. Thoughts about my debt had penetrated my subconscious mind and I was not able to think about anything else. I had seen people with huge credit card or other kinds of debt, but they looked relaxed and comfortable. I wasn't like that. I always paid my bills and rent on time, or even earlier many times. I was not comfortable with this huge debt I had accumulated.

I thought a lot about possible ways to increase my income, but I couldn't come up with a single idea.

By November 2019, I was still thinking of ways to cut my expenses so I could take care of some of my debt, but I still couldn't figure out what to do. In my mind, I was spending my money wisely and there was no room to cut down expenses. A few days passed and another idea hit me: What if I didn't renew my apartment's yearly lease when it came up and moved in with my parents? My parents and sibling had been renting a townhouse, which had an empty basement.

I would be able to save more than $1,000 a month just by leaving my own apartment and moving into my parents' basement. It wasn't a perfect solution—I liked living in my studio apartment because of the sunlight and fresh air, and the basement felt stuffy and dark most of the time. However, I believe in sacrificing short-term comforts and pleasures for long-term improvement, and I was happy to pay the price.

I Was Debt-Free by March 31, 2021

It took me 15 months to pay off my whole debt. I saved a total of $15,600 over that period by living in a stuffy and dark basement. I felt relieved from that huge burden. It was such a freeing feeling. I felt really good about myself. All the investment of money and time I made during the past seven years had paid off.

The Challenge of COVID-19

COVID-19 was another major challenge I was faced with during the entire 2020 year and even the first half of 2021. Although COVID-19 was the global pandemic all of us faced collectively, I was facing unique, individual challenges based on my circumstances. IT professionals usually had the luxury of doing their job from the comfort of their residences, while I had to be in customers' homes not knowing how safe I was there.

Moreover, it was very tough wearing masks and doing repairs at the same time because I had to be in many awkward positions. Sometimes I would be on my stomach lying on the floor, which was difficult with a mask. I also had to deal with the different ways customers were reacting to the pandemic. Some customers refused to wear masks while I was inside their homes doing repairs, and in such situations I politely and professionally refused to provide service. On the other hand, certain customers were very fearful, asking all sorts of questions before letting me into their homes.

I was, however, in a much better position than most doctors, nurses, and paramedics working in hospitals. I was and am truly grateful for services and sacrifices they made—we all had our individual challenges with the pandemic.

Be Careful, Not Fearful

I dealt with these challenges by developing a motto: Be careful, not fearful. Not only did I develop this motto, but I was also thinking, behaving, and acting accordingly. I was wearing my face mask and sanitizing my hands when necessary but having no fear.

Actually, I had some fear but it was not about me but with regard to family members. "What If I get infected with COVID-19? I could easily give it to my family members." Even that fearful thought was not overwhelming or persistent.

I observed noticeable improvement in the way I was thinking and behaving with customers since April 2020. At the same time, I was happily surprised to see I was earning twice as much as I used to on an hourly basis. It was around that same time period when COVID-19 was spreading fear, death, and destruction all over the globe.

Lessons Learned

It doesn't matter what happens to you—it's how you respond to the challenge. The money and time I invested in myself during all those years was paying off. I came out a stronger person after dealing with these two major challenges in 2020. I doubled my income working the same number of hours.

Awareness Lets You Discover More Techniques and Tools

As you gain more and more awareness and move forward in your journey, you will discover more tools and techniques that will help your body, mind, and quality of life. This is because you become aware of what particular activities, practices, or even food makes you feel good and what doesn't.

There are two easy-to-use methods to manage the mindset that require no hard work or any long-term practice:

1. Music

2. Essential oils

Stimulate Your Mind through Music and Music Videos

There are many ways to stimulate your mind so that it can vibrate on a higher frequency. By doing so you attract anything and everything that exists on a higher frequency, whether it's people, conditions, or circumstances. One of my favorite ways is through music or music videos. The difference is quite obvious since you can only listen to music while you can listen as well as watch music videos. Music can help you acquire the mindset you need at any given moment, provided you know what particular mindset you need at a certain time.

For instance, I listen to calming music in the evening to help me relax, and I listen to stimulating music in the morning to help me focus on work and my job. The difference between music and music videos is you can listen to music while doing other activities, but you have to sit down and watch music videos. I find music videos more effective at certain times because I am using my sense of seeing and sense of listening at the same time.

According to an otolaryngologist at Johns Hopkins, "There are few things that stimulate the brain the way music does. If you want to keep your brain engaged throughout the aging process, listening to or playing music is a great tool. It provides a total brain workout."[51] Research has shown that listening to music can improve anxiety, blood pressure, pain, sleep quality, mood, mental alertness, and memory.[52]

To be more creative, you can listen to any music you like, as we all have our favorite types of music. But if you want to be more creative, listen to new types of music. According to Johns Hopkins, "New music challenges the brain in a way that old music doesn't. It might not feel pleasurable at first, but that unfamiliarity forces the brain to struggle to understand the new sound."[53]

I watch Bollywood films and music videos on YouTube in the morning because watching beautiful actresses and scenery with music behind them really stimulates me. There are countless Hindi music videos from the '80s, '90s and 2000s that I like to watch. However, I usually don't watch music videos in the evening. Instead, I practice meditation by putting on headphones and listening to CDs on my laptop.

Managing My Mood Using Essentials Oils

I discovered the benefits of essentials oils in two ways. First, I learned from newsletters I got from an online health product website called VitaCost.com. Second, I watched a webinar from a company called Aromatics International. The process of discovery was rather slow.

The company Nicole Rose Studio describes essential oils the following way: "Essential oils are compounds extracted from plants. The oils capture the plant's scent and flavor, or 'essence.' Unique aromatic compounds give each essential oil its characteristic essence. Essential oils are obtained through distillation or mechanical methods, such as cold pressing. Once the aromatic chemicals have been extracted, they are combined with a carrier oil to create a product that's ready for use."[54]

I started using essential oils and found out that they helped me generate positive moods and emotions. Essential oils are said to help with many medical conditions, although I mostly use them to promote sleep. I put drops of lavender oil on my pillow before bedtime and it promotes better sleep. I also use lavender oil to calm myself if I get excited, anxious, or upset by putting drops on a small piece of fabric and keeping it over my nose for five to fifteen minutes.

According to registered dietician Helen West, "Inhaling the aromas from essential oils can stimulate areas of your limbic system, which is a part of your brain that plays a role in emotions, behaviors, sense of smell, and long-term memory."[55]

Lessons Learned

I went through a lot of discomfort from two major challenges in 2020. However, I turned these challenges into opportunities and made the year one of the most productive of my life. Moreover, I learned two tools and modalities to manage my feelings and moods.

CHAPTER 8

The Process of
My Transformation

The Process of My Transformation

I am going to summarize the steps I took during my personal growth journey in an organized form for you to understand and follow. Here is the six-step process that I went through:

Step 1: It all started with asking myself the three important questions Bob Proctor asked

1. What do I want to have, to do, and to be? Not what I think I can achieve, but really want to have, to do and to be. Keep in mind your wants may change as you grow to become a higher person. I started out wanting mostly material things, but my wants changed from material things to fulfillment and joy. But you still have to ask this question.

2. Am I able to achieve my goals? We are spiritual beings living in physical bodies and as such we have infinite potential within us. So, if you can see the truth, then the answer would clearly be "Yes."

3. Am I willing to pay the price? This is the most important question you need to ask yourself. We all want to live a happy, healthy, and wealthy life, but not all of us want to pay the price that needs to be paid before we can live our dream life. If you are willing to pay the price, then you have to make the committed decision in your heart as well in writing.

Step 2: Decision

Napoleon Hill writes about decisions in his book *Think and Grow Rich*: "People who achieve success have the habit of reaching decisions promptly and of changing them slowly, if and when they were changed."[56] Moreover, you have to make decisions from where you are with whatever you have. That is why most people cannot make decisions—they always let present circumstances control their decisions.

Step 3: Raise awareness

You must raise your level of awareness. You simply cannot achieve your goals from your current level of awareness. There are many ways to increase your level of awareness.

1. Read inspirational books that align with and support your goals. Reading books essentially means self-study. I would recommend having a mentor, either online or in-person, at least initially. But if you decided to go this path, then you have to read books mindfully, giving yourself permission to read them again and again if necessary to understand the lessons the books teach.

2. Enroll in personnel growth programs. There are many online and in-person programs you can enroll in (I have mentioned the programs I participated in). You will receive

some support in this route. You can also attend seminars and they can give good value. Although most participants get really excited after attending the seminars, they easily go back to old ways of being and thinking. Thus, it is important to commit to implementing at least one action step from whatever resonated most from the seminar attended, as baby steps lead to larger steps.

Step 4: Develop six faculties of mind

You also raise your awareness by developing your faculties of mind. Most people live their lives through their five senses. Humans are the most evolved beings on earth. The six faculties of mind are marvelous tools, which can help us to achieve success and happiness in life.

We must develop the following six faculties of mind in order to achieve higher objectives in our lives.

1. **Reason**

   Reason is simply logical or sensible thinking. Reason is in opposition of sensation and feeling. Reason is the capacity of consciously applying logic to seek truth and draw conclusions.

2. **Will**

   The ability to focus on only one idea and exclude everything else. Will gives us an ability to stay focused on our goals.

3. **Perception**

   Two people can be looking at the same thing and can have different ideas about what they see. In other words, they perceive things differently. In this instance, there is no right or wrong. They are merely different points of views.

4. **Memory**

   The mental faculty that helps us retain and revise facts, events, and impressions. It can also be used for recalling or recognizing previous experiences.

5. **Intuition**

   Intuition provides us with a direct perception of truth and fact independent of any reasoning factors. It can also be defined as an instant idea or immediate answer we receive without even thinking about it.

6. **Imagination**

   It has been said that we can create anything we can imagine. Napoleon Hill writes about the imagination, "The impulse, the desire, is given shape, form and action through the aid of imaginative faculty of mind."[57]

Step 5: Set goals beyond your comfort zone

You need to set goals that are beyond your comfort zone because that's how you grow. Start with what you really want and set goals that really excite and scare you at the same time. Goals give you a target to start moving toward something you want.

As Bob Proctor said, "Change is inevitable, but personal growth is a choice."[58]

Step 6: Discovery process

If you truly set goals beyond your comfort zone, it is likely that you will fail to achieve your goals on your first attempt. Failure gives you an opportunity to start the discovery process. In the discovery process not only can you learn the mistakes you made, but also about you, your beliefs, and your behaviors.

Once you learn from your mistakes as well as learn about yourself, then you can go back to start working on your goals.

After investing money, time, and effort in my personal growth journey for more than two years, I decided to set a goal that was beyond my comfort zone. I decided to double my income by building an online business. I was really excited and scared while setting this goal. I had no idea how I would achieve it. I just took a leap of faith.

Building My Online Business

In November 2017, I came to notice so many people from all over the world with no business experience were hitting the jackpot by launching products on Amazon. I was so excited about this opportunity that I bought an online specialized training specifically designed for the Amazon platform from Rapid Crush. This training taught me almost all aspects from searching products to sourcing products to launching products to advertising products all on Amazon.

After searching for a product, I decided to launch Pain Massager Kit as my first product. One of the most important parts of launching a successful business at Amazon was doing a lot of research to finding the right products that suit individual sellers' needs. There were so many criteria to be considered, such as price range for a single unit, weight of the product (the heavier the weight the more the shipping cost), size of the product (larger products incur higher shipping costs), competition (how many sellers are in this product category), among other factors.

I thought it would be easy to sell these Pain Massager Kits, since nobody was selling them at the time. I based my criteria on that single factor. I sourced a quality product, had attractive images professionally made, and had a brand logo printed on tote bags, which I specially designed for the massager kit. I invested money on an advertising campaign. I gave the best I possibly could at the time.

I launched my product the way I was taught, but I wasn't able to sell a single unit the first week. I tried different ways to improve my business for six months, but at the end I failed miserably. Unfortunately, I didn't do the right research on finding the right product. I was disappointed, but I didn't want to give up. I took a break for a month to get my mind off the failure.

After that break, I did more product research and chose a baby pillow to be my next product. Baby Pillow for Newborn was a better product for many reasons, one of which was that the average selling price for the baby pillow was $15, compared to the Pain Massager Kit's selling price of $45. Moreover, there was much more demand for the baby pillow. I invested money on searching tools too.

Baby Pillow was designed to keep a newborn's head in a proper shape. I achieved some initial success and sold 500 units, although it took eight months to achieve that. I placed another order of five hundred baby pillows to be shipped from a wholesaler to Amazon. There were so many sellers starting to sell the same kind of baby pillow that by the time my inventory arrived at Amazon's fulfillment center the market was saturated, and I barely sold 100 units. I lost a considerable sum of money in unsold inventory, advertising, and other costs.

After careful consideration, I decided to close down my online business. Not only because I lost money but also because I suffered business failure. Naturally I was disappointed and sad. I decided to find out why I kept failing. If I were to succeed in any business,

I would have to find out the reasons of my failure. I started my discovery process.

I committed to writing a journal at least three times a week. It was my first step in the discovery process.

Journal Writing

I would write in my journal from time to time and found it to be an effective tool. For example, I used to journal to communicate with myself. Also, I used to journal to look at certain issues from different angles. I started free flow writing about the possible causes of my business failures. I was asking my mind questions such as "What were the mistakes I possibly made?"

I wasn't able to find any real causes of my failure in business endeavors. I decided to continue my discovery process and go much deeper, but I had no idea what my next step should be. Nature shows the next step if you are committed.

The Hoffman Process, Class of August 2019

I was determined to find the answer with regard to why I was failing in my business endeavors. No matter what price I had to pay. I found out about the Hoffman Process through the personal growth webinar I attended by Natalie Ledwell (cofounder of Mind Movies).[59] She was sharing her personal growth journey and how she was transformed by the process. I also did my online research by going through people's testimonials and transformation stories. I was impressed with what I found out.

I didn't have the funds to participate in the Hoffman Process, because I already had credit card and student loan debt. But I was determined to participate anyway. Luckily, I got a Hoffman grant covering 30 percent of the cost, which I discussed earlier.

The process revealed who I was. I became aware of my beliefs, patterns, and behaviors. Not only was I able to find out about my negative beliefs, patterns, and behaviors, but I was able to release some of them as well. I was also given tools and techniques to work on my remaining negative patterns, beliefs, and behaviors. There was a long list, but let me share some of them with you to help you understand what I mean:

- Indecisive

- Jealousy/envy

- Fatalism/why bother

- Self-sabotage

- Feeling and acting like a victim

In some of the therapies I tried, I hadn't been able to come up with a decisive list of my negative thoughts, beliefs, and behaviors. None of the therapists I'd seen had given me the tools to identify them or overcome them, but the Hoffman Process succeeded where they failed. It got me thinking about those things before I even attended the retreat by having me fill out a lot of personal questionnaires that dug deep into myself.

By filling those out on my own, I really had to think about the answers and it started an incredible self-discovery process before I'd even gone to the retreat. I went into the program feeling more aware of what I needed to work on for my personal circumstances rather than just taking the one-size-fits-all steps I'd encountered in other programs.

What Is the Hoffman Process All About?

You might be wondering why the hell I spent lots of money (total cost was around $5,000 for tuition, lodging, and meals) on the Hoffman Process when I could have received countless sessions with any kind of psychotherapist for the same cost. Well, there is huge difference between psychotherapy of any kind and the Hoffman Process retreat.

Most therapies involve talking to work through problems and dig deep. Therapists help guide you to your problems and resolve them. It is more focused on mental and emotional health.

The Hoffman Process starts by getting you to identify your own problems before you even go on the retreat. It starts with paperwork long before you meet in person by having you answer questions about yourself, your parents, your childhood, and your relationship with your parents. The Hoffman Process is not about dealing with mental or emotional diseases but raising awareness.

Awareness is not the same as knowing about something. It's about watching to see how you create certain results as you create them, meaning:

- How you feel

- How you behave

- Which people and situations you attract or become attracted to

- What meanings you assign to the events in your life

You have no choice or control over what you're unaware of. However, you gain choice over it once you become aware of it. It is about consciously creating your circumstances, controlling your environment, and building the life you want. You can't do any of that if you aren't first aware of yourself, your needs and wants, your actions and reactions, etc.

Awareness creates choice. I gained awareness not only about my beliefs, my patterns and behaviors, but also how and why I acquired them. However, I still had the challenge of how not react to certain patterns. As I said, healing and growth are a journey.[60]

The Hoffman Quadrinity Process, founded by Bob Hoffman in 1967, is a week-long residential and personal growth retreat that helps participants identify negative behaviors, moods, and ways of thinking that developed unconsciously and were developed in childhood. The process helps you become conscious of and disconnected from negative patterns of thought and behaviors on an emotional, intellectual, physical, and spiritual level in order to make significant positive changes in your life. It teaches you how to remove habitual ways of thinking and behaving, align with your authentic self, and respond to situations in your life from a place of conscious choice—a place that is constructive rather than self-destructive.

When I went to the Hoffman retreat, it was me and 31 strangers together for a week. It was really awkward at first, especially since I felt like they were all so much more successful than I was, but we are all there for the same reason. We needed guidance.

The 32 of us were split into four groups and there were four teachers working with us. We did a lot of unique exercises to get us to think about ourselves, but also about how we impacted the world and people around us. In one exercise we had to write our own eulogies. It was so we could take a look at what we would be remembered for and how other people saw us.

Another day, we just played a bunch of group games. Loosening up, engaging with strangers, and having fun together was a great way to learn how to have positive interactions with strangers.

It wasn't just a lecture or an online course—the entire retreat was interactive.

One of my greatest limiting beliefs before the retreat was that I was a victim. I felt like everything was always working against me. Part of the program required us to take a look at our beliefs and see how they were influencing us. My belief was that I was a victim. I thought that circumstances were always working against me and I was powerless to change them. Throughout my time at the Hoffman retreat, I had to revisit this again and again, and I finally had to outgrow that mindset. I realized I wasn't a victim caught up in everyone else's messes. I had the choice to take charge and be the person I wanted to be and to have the interactions I wanted to have.

It was because of this realization and awareness that I began to have better interactions with my customers, leading to me doubling my income and actually feeling happy about my job. Just a small shift in my thought process, and my entire life turned around!

In a 2006 journal article, the Hoffman Process was shown to have outstanding results. Program participants demonstrated significant and lasting increases in emotional intelligence, forgiveness, compassion, life satisfaction and vitality, coupled with significant and lasting decreases in depression, hostility, and anxiety.[61]

Lessons Learned

I discovered my mental blocks were the real reasons for my failure in my business endeavor. Although I lost a lot of money, time, and effort during my business endeavor, I learned who I really was and what I was capable of. I learned that I was not a failure, even though I failed at my business endeavor. The more awareness you gain, the better your life becomes. This is because you discover more and more techniques to manage your feeling, moods, and behavior.

Although I grew during the whole process of raising awareness, setting goals, building my business, and the discovery process, I developed sleep issues.

The Challenge of Getting Quality Sleep

I got really stressed out in the process of building my online business because I had been facing failure after failure. Yes, I grew as an individual, but it took a heavy toll on my mind and body and my problem of waking up in the middle of the night got worse. I started waking up three times a night due to nighttime urination, since my bladder gets really affected from stress.

I wasn't able to get six to eight hours of quality sleep. Lack of sleep caused me to be moody, irritable, and angry. I couldn't think with clarity and I couldn't focus on anything. I had a hard time doing my job. I realized just how important sleep was. As a result I did research on different aspects of sleep, such as why getting quality sleep is important, the price we pay if we don't get quality sleep and why we sleep.

Why Do We Sleep?

The effects of quality sleep are well-documented. Dr. John Bigelow states, "The results of my studies have not only strengthened my convictions that supposed exemption from customary toils and activities was not the final purpose of sleep, but have also made clearer to my mind the conviction that no part of man's life deserves to be considered more indispensable to its symmetrical and perfect spiritual development than the while he is separated from the phenomenal world of sleep."[62]

Detrimental Effects of Lack of Sleep

Soomi Lee, assistant professor in the School of Aging Studies at the University of South Florida, found that "…the biggest jump in symptoms appeared after just one night of sleep loss. The number of mental and physical problems steadily got worse, peaking on day three. At that point, research shows the human body got relatively used to repeated sleep loss. But that all changed on day six, when participants reported that the severity of physical symptoms was at its worst."[63]

I saw a urologist in 2007 while living in Flagstaff, AZ and took medications for a few months to relax the bladder muscles so urine can pass more easily. However, I didn't believe in taking any medication for long-term. I wanted a holistic solution.

I saw a physical therapist who specialized in the pelvic floor in early 2021, and she helped me with daytime as well as nighttime urination issues, including urgency and frequency, by using various techniques and exercises, including Kegel and Reverse Kegel exercises.

I also combined these techniques and exercises with pumpkin-based dietary supplements and the results were awesome—meaning I didn't wake up in the middle of night to go to the bathroom, or just once a night. However, when I got stressed out, my bladder, being the weakest organ, gets stressed out as well, and I have to wake twice a night all over again. I had to teach myself better practices for maintaining quality sleep.

Here is how I practice maintaining quality sleep:

- **Stay away from electronic devices at night.**

  I don't scroll through social media, watch videos, or read news articles right before going to bed, since it can really affect my sleep in a negative way. The blue light emitted from electronic devices disrupts the production of melatonin, the brain chemical that makes you feel tired and puts you to sleep.

- **Sunshine helps.**

  I get more sunshine during the day whenever I can. Natural sunshine has been shown to improve sleep quality and duration in those with insomnia by improving your Vitamin D intake. Natural sunlight helps the brain establish the right chemical production for proper sleep and wake cycles when there is so much unnatural light that can confuse the brain.

- **Healthy diet choices can help with sleep.**

  I avoid having sugary foods as well as caffeinated and alcoholic drinks in the evening. Not only does consuming sugary food and drink right before bed lead to weight gain, it also makes it harder to sleep thanks to the sugar rush that follows. The same goes for caffeinated beverages such as soda, coffee, and tea. Caffeine can stay in your body for up to six hours after your last drink, and it blocks the receptors in your brain from feeling tired. Alcohol can cause all sorts of problems. Not only does it impact the melatonin our body produces naturally, but it also increases instances of sleep apnea, snoring, and restless sleep.

- **The timing of dinner is important.**

  I find the timing of dinner affects my sleep. Therefore, I eat my dinner usually three hours prior to bedtime. If I go to bed too early or right after dinner, then it is harder for me to sleep on a full stomach. On the other hand, if I go to bed too late after having dinner, then I might feel hungry in the middle of the night.

- **Evening walk.**

  I walk 20 to 30 minutes, usually before dinner. Don't walk right after dinner. Allow two hours to pass by if you choose to walk after dinner. It elevates your mood and reduces stress.

- **Sleep environment is important.**

  I make sure I am in a quiet and relaxing environment. I never let my room get too cold or too hot, especially hot. I keep it dark.

- **Reduce my stress any way I can.**

  There are so many ways to reduce stress levels before going to bed. I sometimes put drops of lavender essential oil on my pillow. I sometimes read a book or soak in a bathtub with Epsom salt and drops of essential oils for 20 minutes.

Lessons Learned

I am glad I went through all of those business failures, monetary losses, disappointment, and suffering, because I came out to be a better and stronger person. I was ready to pay the price and I did.

CHAPTER 9

Transformation in Action

Transformation in Action

I **discovered** my purpose—to share the wisdom independently with others from the peacefulness I find in nature—in August 2021. Why is discovering my purpose so important and what does it do for me?

We all have specific talents and gifts given to us. It is essential that we find out what are we good at and what we love doing. I was wandering aimlessly. Now my purpose guides my ambitions, vision, and goals.

I used to get a sense of satisfaction from fixing appliances, until 2017. Now I feel disgusted with this new trend of appliances breaking down without the prospect of being repaired at a reasonable cost.

Appliance Industry and the Importance of Right Thinking

In my experience, appliances used to last 30-plus years on an average. Nowadays major appliance brands tend to break down on average after a three-year period, and half the time the repair cost is prohibitive.

For instance, if a compressor dies in three years in certain LG refrigerators, the compressor replacement is not cost effective. And if the wash motor starts leaking water after three years in certain Whirlpool dishwashers, again replacing it with a new wash motor doesn't make sense.

I have to let customers know that sometimes it is better to buy a new appliance than to repair their current one because of the cost. I can go on and on. If you were to start replacing your washing machine, dryer, refrigerator, oven, range, and dishwasher every three years, it adds to lots of money.

We have made tremendous achievements in technology over the years. Why is it that we have made so much advancement in agriculture, food, and medical technology, and yet society is only able to manage diseases instead of curing them?

I can go on and on.

As a matter of fact, we have made tremendous achievements in almost every field including biology, physics, robotics, chemistry, computers, smart phones, and aviation. We are at the crossroads of human civilization. Now we need to focus on human thinking and make sure that human beings can think right.

It is up to us as a collective society to begin pursuing our own health, happiness, and wealth in order to improve our own lives, but also to improve global society. That is the crossroads we are at. By living your happiest, healthiest life, it creates a ripple effect to the people around you.

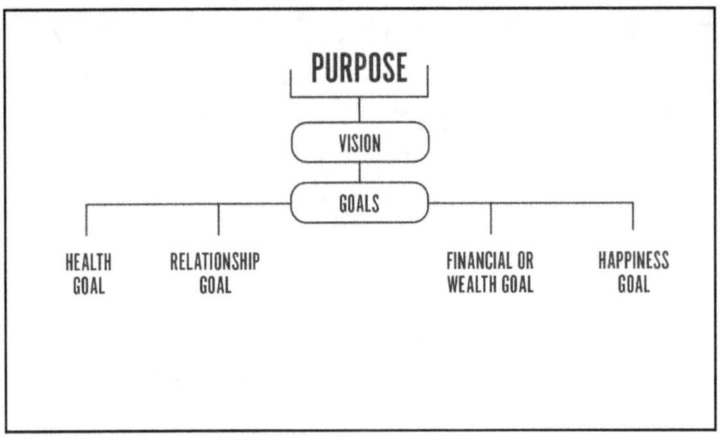

We all have a unique purpose and we need to discover our purpose—that is what we love to do. Purpose leads to vision and vision leads to goals. Once you discover your purpose you have to create and maintain a vision to express that purpose. Vision is the strategy behind the fulfillment of your purpose. You accomplish this strategy by creating goals.

My Desire for You

I took my personal growth journey because I was sick of being sick. I was tired of feeling angry and unhappy. I was miserable from being miserable. Put bluntly, I was forced to start my journey. I started to experience small shifts in less than a year while I was in my personal growth journey and that was enough to keep me motivated. I am glad I took the journey.

Are you feeling miserable or you are somewhat happy and somewhat healthy? If you are miserable, may it be your physical health or mental health or even marital life, you have nothing to lose but your misery and suffering. So, go ahead and start following suggestions with whatever resonates with you in this book.

You will be glad you did.

On the other hand, if you are living a somewhat happy and healthy life, then you may not be finding enough motivation. You may find it hard to come out from your comfort zone. But I urge you to try, because you will be glad you did after enjoying your results. You will be more productive and focused. You will be happier and healthier. I wish you good luck and urge you to take even small steps, but on a consistent basis. The key is consistency.

This is the only life you've got—so far as we know—so make the best of it.

Acknowledgments

I have to start by thanking my mother Talat Siddiqui for loving me and making sacrifices for me. She played an important role in my life despite the fact that she lacked a high level of awareness. As such, I dare to write this book only because the way I am.

I also have to thank Tracey Renee Mckee who happens to be my Reiki Master. She was the first person who read my first manuscript and fell in love with it. She encouraged me to move forward with this project.

Writing a book appears to be an individual project, but the reality is that if you want to write a great book, it takes an entire team. I would like to thank everyone on my publishing team.

Finally, I am deeply grateful to all the people, such as my personal growth teacher, hypnotherapist and psychotherapist, who helped me heal and grow to become who I am now.

Endnotes

1   "Stress Effects on the Body," American Psychological Association, November 1, 2018, https://www.apa.org/topics/stress/body.

2   Debra Fulghum Bruce, "Symptoms of Depression," WebMD, September 17, 2021, https://www.webmd.com/depression/guide/detecting-depression.

3   Ibid.

4   "Depression: How effective are antidepressants?" NCBI, updated June 18, 2020, https://www.ncbi.nlm.nih.gov/books/NBK361016/.

5   Ibid.

6   Nancy Schimelpfening, "Can Antidepressants Cure Depression?" Verywell Mind,

7   Kelly Miller, "27 Scientifically Proven Benefits of Counseling," Positive Psychology, November 2, 2022, https://positivepsychology.com/benefits-of-counseling/.

8   "Potential Benefits of Counseling," Coe College, accessed March 3, 2022, https://www.coe.edu/student-life/student-life-resources/health-wellness/mental-health-counseling/potential-benefits-counseling.

9   "7 Types of Mental Health Therapy," Healthily, February 18, 2019, https://www.livehealthily.com/mental-health-therapy.

10   Saul McLeod, "Cognitive Behavioral Therapy (CBT)," Simply Psychology, updated 2019, https://www.simplypsychology.org/cognitive-therapy.html.

11   "Hypnotherapy," Cleveland Clinic, October 7, 2019, https://my.clevelandclinic.org/health/treatments/9930-hypnotherapy.

12   Ibid.

13   Smitha Bhandari, "Mental Health and Hypnosis," WebMD, September 14, 2021, https://www.webmd.com/mental-health/mental-health-hypnotherapy.

14   "EMDR," The Other Road Counseling, accessed March 3, 2022, https://theotherroadcounseling.com/emdr-therapy/.

15   Salynn Boyles, "Dietary Supplement Ups Antidepressant Effect," WebMD, December 2, 2004, https://www.webmd.com/depression/news/20041202/dietary-supplement-ups-antidepressant-effect.

16   Ibid.

17   Huijeong Ahn, Jeeyoung Kim, Min-Jae Lee, Young Jin Kim, Young-Wook Cho, and Geun-Shik Lee, "Methylsulfonylmethane Inhibits NLRP3 Inflammasome Activation," PubMed.gov, February 2015, https://pubmed.ncbi.nlm.nih.gov/25461402/.

18   "Dietary and Herbal Supplements," National Center for Complementary and Integrative Medicine, updated February 2020, https://www.nccih.nih.gov/health/dietary-and-herbal-supplements.

19   Mary Jane Brown, "Synthetic vs. Natural Nutrients: Does It Matter?" Healthline, August 17, 2016, https://www.healthline.com/nutrition/synthetic-vs-natural-nutrients.

20   Ibid.

21   Ibid.

22   Ibid.

23   Jennifer M. Granholn, 2006 Economic Report of the Governor, transmitted to the Michigan Legislature, December 2006, https://www.michigan.gov/documents/taxes/2006EconReportGov_181443_7.pdf.

24   "Cognitive Behavioral Therapy," Mayo Clinic, accessed February 16, 2022, https://www.mayoclinic.org/tests-procedures/cognitive-behavioral-therapy/about/pac-20384610.

25   Allison Aubrey, "Forest Bathing: A Retreat to Nature Can Boost Immunity and Mood," NPR, July 17, 2017, https://www.npr.org/sections/health-shots/2017/07/17/536676954/forest-bathing-a-retreat-to-nature-can-boost-immunity-and-mood.

26   Bob Proctor, You Were Born Rich: Now You Can Discover and Develop Those Riches (Scottsdale: LifeSuccess Productions, 1997).

27   Margaret M. Hansen, Reo Jones, and Kirsten Tocchini, "Shinrin-Yoku (Forest Bathing) and Nature: A State-of-the-Art Review," International Journal of Environmental Research and Public Health 8, no. 4 (August 2017): 851, https://www.doi.org/10.3390/ijerph14080851.

28   StarBasil, "Phytoncides: The Science Behind Forest Bathing Benefits," Forest Bathing Central, December 8, 2020, https://forestbathingcentral.com/phytoncides/.

29   "Controlling Anger," Pediatric Psychology Associates, accessed March 3, 2022, https://www.southfloridatherapists.com/areas-of-specialty/controlling-anger/#:~:text=Anger%20is%20an%20emotional%20state,energy%20hormones%2C%20adrenalin%20and%20noradrenalin.

30   "Understanding Anger," @Health, October 23, 2013, https://athealth.com/topics/understanding-anger-2/#:~:text=People%20often%20confuse%20anger%20with,not%20necessarily%20lead%20to%20aggression.

31   Corrina Horne, "What is Maladaptive Behavior? Definition and Symptoms," Betterhelp, updated February 1,2022, https://www.betterhelp.com/advice/behavior/what-is-maladaptive-behavior-definition-and-symptoms/.

32   Patrick M. Reilly, Michael S. Shopshire, Timothy C. Durazzo, and Torri A. Campbell, Anger Management for Substance Abuse and Mental Health Clients—Participant Workbook, Updated 2019 (Rockville: SAMHSA, 2019), 22, https://store.samhsa.gov/sites/default/files/d7/priv/anger_management_workbook_508_compliant.pdf.

33   Ibid.

34   Ibid.

35   Ibid.

36   "4 Types of Communication Styles," Alvernia University, March 27, 2018, https://online.alvernia.edu/articles/4-types-communication-styles/#:~:text=Every%20person%20has%20a%20unique,and%20why%20individuals%20use%20them.

37   Bob Proctor, The ABCs of Success: The Essential Principles from America's Greatest Prosperity Teacher (New York: Jeremy P. Tarcher/Penguin), 183.

38   Bob Proctor, "Understanding the Power of Paradigms," April 21, 2016, YouTube video, https://www.youtube.com/watch?v=XOe6ZCYWHZ8.

39   Bob Proctor, "Six Minutes to Success," Proctor Gallagher Institute, accessed February 17, 2022, https://www.proctorgallagherinstitute.com/programs/6-minutes-to-success.

40   Bob Proctor Coaching, Proctor Gallagher Institute, accessed February 17, 2022, https://www.proctorgallagherinstitute.com/programs/coaching.

41   Proctor

42   , You Were Born Rich.

irected by James Colquhoun, Laurentine Ten Bosch, and Carlo Ledesma (Brisbane: Permacology Productions, 2012).

43   Forks over Knives, directed by Lee Fulkerson (Santa Monica: Monica Beach Media, 2011).

44   "What is Epigenetics?" Centers for Disease Control and Prevention, updated August 3, 2020, https://www.cdc.gov/genomics/disease/epigenetics.htm#:~:text=Epigenetics%20is%20the%20study%20of,body%20reads%20a%20DNA%20sequence.

45   Carter Lewis, "Is Your Diet Changing Your DNA?" The Good Kitchen, accessed March 4, 2022, https://www.thegoodkitchen.com/blogs/the-good-kitchen-blog/is-your-diet-changing-your-dna.

46   "About," Dr. Hyman, accessed March 4, 2022, https://drhyman.com/about/.

47   Melissa Groves, "7 Great Reasons to Add Sprouted Bread to Your Diet," Healthline, June 20, 2018,

48   Cara Rosenbloom, "Sugar, Fiber, Pasteurization: Here's What You Need to Know About Juice," the Washington Post, August 7, 2019, https://www.washingtonpost.com/lifestyle/wellness/can-juice-be-part-of-a-healthy-diet-maybe-but-its-better-to-eat-whole-produce-instead/2019/08/06/8ae10a88-b795-11e9-a091-6a96e67d9cce_story.html.

49   Marcus Aurelius, Meditations, trans. Martin Hammond (New York: Penguin, 2006).

50   "What Is the Hoffman Process?" Hoffman, accessed March 4, 2022, https://www.hoffmaninstitute.org/the-process/.

51   "Keep Your Brain Young with Music," Johns Hopkins Medicine, accessed February 17, 2022, https://www.hopkinsmedicine.org/health/wellness-and-prevention/keep-your-brain-young-with-music.

52   Ibid.

53   Ibid.

54   "Essential Oil 101," Nicole Rose Studio, March 27, 2020, https://www.nicolerosestudio.com/blog/2020/3/27/what-are-essential-oils-and-how-do-they-work.

55   Helen West, "What Are Essential Oils, and Do They Work?" Healthline, September 30, 2019, https://www.healthline.com/nutrition/what-are-essential-oils#:~:text=Inhaling%20the%20aromas%20from%20essential,heavily%20involved%20in%20forming%20memories.

56   Napoleon Hill, Think and Grow Rich (New York: Jeremy P. Tarcher/Penguin, 2003).

57   Ibid.

58   Bob Proctor, Facebook, November 9, 2019, https://www.facebook.com/OfficialBobProctor/photos/change-is-inevitable-but-personal-growth-is-a-choicewhen-

you-change-your-perspec/10157831857024421/.

59   Natalie Ledwell personal website, accessed February 17, 2022, https://www.natalieledwell.com/.

60   Bill Harris, The New Science of Raising Awareness: Use the Newest Brain Science Discoveries to Create Astonishing Levels of Awareness, Zen-Like Meditation, Happiness, Intelligence, Creativity, Motivation, and Flow (Beaverton: Centerpointe Research Institute, 2015).

61   Michael R. Levinson, Carolyn M. Aldwin, and Loriena Yancura, "Positive Emotional Change: Mediating Effects of Forgiveness and Spirituality," Explore: The Journal of Science and Healing 2 (2006): 498-508, https://www.doi.org/10.1016/j.explore.2006.08.002.

62   Joseph Murphey, The Power of Your Subconscious Mind (Mansfield Centre: Martino Publishing, 2011).

63   "Drama Llama or Sleep Deprived? New Study Uncovers How Consistent Sleep Loss Impacts Mental and Physical Well-being," University of South Florida, July 6, 2021, https://www.usf.edu/news/2021/drama-llama-or-sleep-deprived-new-study-uncovers-sleep-loss-impacts-mental-and-physical-well-being.aspx.

TAKE A STEP
TODAY

How can you focus on losing weight and getting your body physically healthy while also spending your time trying to train your mind to think more positively? To find out more, go to **suicidaltoserene.com**.

Order discounted bulk purchases of the book for your organization or community:
Elk House Publishing
elkhousepublishing@gmail.com

Book Amir Siddiqui for podcast interviews and speaking at **suicidaltoserene.com**.

GET MORE INSIGHTS AND STAY UP TO DATE ON FUTURE PROJECTS BY FOLLOWING AMIR ON SOCIAL MEDIA

@Let's grow to be happy and healthy

@amirsiddiqui337

THANK YOU FOR READING!

Thank you for reading! If you enjoyed *From Suicidal to Serene*, please leave a review on Goodreads, Amazon, or retailer site where you purchased this book.

www.ingramcontent.com/pod-product-compliance
Lightning Source LLC
Chambersburg PA
CBHW071328150726
47997CB00002B/634